NUTRIBULLET
RECIPE BOOK

100 Green Smoothie Recipes

---

for
weight loss, detox, & vitality.

By
Kate Billington

Disclaimer

It is important to note, before making any of the recipes contained in this book, you should first contact your health practitioner or GP with regard to following a healthy lifestyle. Some recipes contain nuts and seeds, and should therefore be avoided by those suffering from nut allergies.

All instructions and safety advice provided by your machine should be read thoroughly before proceeding with recipe making.

This book is written to supplement the Nutribullet and is in no way affiliated with Nutribullet LLC. Nutribullet LLC was not involved in any of the recipe experimenting and developing, and is not affiliated with any of the recipes in this book.

First published August 2015

ISBN-13: 978-1517084523

ISBN-10: 1517084520

CONTENTS

....

INTRODUCTION

....

T he Nutribullet has become synonymous with health and wellbeing over the last couple of years. Since its introduction not so long ago, people have transformed their diets, becoming healthier, fitter, and skinnier. Not only this, but they have introduced more fruit and vegetables into their daily lives, much more than they were eating before.

This wonderful invention is not only simple to use but it takes 2 minutes to clean, what could be better than that! There are so many recipes to come up with, with so many healthy, colourful, nutritious ingredients to choose from.

The Nutribullet works by extracting all of the nutrients from the ingredients used, even ingredients such as hard-to-digest leafy greens. This ensures the digestive system can more easily absorb the precious nutrients that may otherwise be lost from other forms of blending. As a result, our body is provided with a form of nutrition that ensures healthy cell production, a healthy cardiovascular system, increased energy levels, a strong immune system, protection against free radical damage, and an efficient digestive system.

Nutribullet smoothies are empowering; they provide a quick and efficient pathway to a healthier lifestyle, one that can be easily maintained and managed. Whether you want a smoothie for breakfast, lunch, dinner, or just as a healthy snack, the Nutribullet provides you with everything you need to get started.

Enjoy!

CHAPTER ONE
Green Smoothies & Their Benefits

Green smoothies are a mixture of green vegetables and fruit, blended together to create a healthy drink full of essential nutrients. Not many people like to eat bowls of leafy greens or large plates of green vegetables because, a) they don't like the taste, or b) they don't have enough time to prepare them.

The introduction of green smoothies to your diet eliminates both of these problems because the taste of the greens can easily be masked by adding tasty fruits such as apple, mango or pineapple, plus the preparation time is minimal, just wash and chop!

Green smoothies are also a clever way to trick your kids into eating their greens! Make sure there is plenty of sweet fruit added and watch them grow healthy and strong.

Probably the most important factor to consider about green smoothies is the fact that you are eating raw ingredients. Greens that have been cooked lose a lot of valuable vitamins and minerals, making them less nutrient dense. Also, greens are high in cellulose which makes them difficult for the digestive system to break down. Mixing the greens in a blender, particularly a Nutribullet, breaks the cellulose down, making the nutrients more easily absorbed by our cells.

Just some of the positive effects of drinking green smoothies include;

- an improved cardiovascular system.

- clearer skin.

- improved collagen production in the skin.

- the elimination of digestive disorders such as constipation and IBS.

- increased energy levels.

- increased healthy weight loss.

- a strong immune system.

- healthy bone density.

- a lower risk of disease.

- promotes a good night's sleep.

- reduces inflammation in the skin.

- anti-aging.

CHAPTER TWO
Vitamins, Minerals, & Antioxidants

V itamins play a vital role in the health and vitality of our body. Unfortunately however, most Western diets today are high in saturated fats, red meat and sugary carbohydrates while being low in fresh fruits, vegetables and whole grains. This ultimately leads to a deficiency in one or more important vitamins, which can cause lowered energy levels, colds and flu, various diseases and disorders, early signs of aging and a sluggish digestive system.

Thankfully, the addition of healthy smoothies in your daily life is a fantastic way to meet and exceed your dietary need for essential vitamins. The most important vitamins found in the smoothie recipes contained in this book are outlined in more detail below;

Vitamin A
This is an essential vitamin for our skin and immune system, supporting the overall health of the skin, while helping to fight off infection and disease. Protecting and preserving our eyesight is also another important function. Carrots, spinach, kale, pumpkins and peaches are excellent sources.

Beta Carotene
Also known as pro-vitamin A, beta carotene is one of the most widely researched carotenoids for a very good reason. It is a powerful antioxidant, helping the body to fight free radicals thereby reducing the damage to cell membranes, protein structures in the cell and DNA. It also has fantastic anti aging and anti cancer properties. Beta carotene is found in abundance in almost all green, yellow and orange

fruits and vegetables including watercress, kale, carrots, collard greens, spinach, watermelon, papaya, oranges and apricots.

Vitamin B
B vitamins are called the happy vitamins as they bring balance to the body, keeping it energetic and healthy. There are actually 8 B vitamins, all of which are essential for metabolism, growth and repair, blood cell formation and a healthy digestive system.

B1 (Thiamin) – Plays an important role in the normal functioning of the nervous system, aids the function of the heart and maintains the formation of red blood cells. Thiamin uses protein, fats and carbohydrates from the food we consume and converts them into energy. Flaxseed, sunflower seeds and oranges contain vitamin B1.

B2 (Riboflavin) – This B vitamin plays a vital role in the body's energy production. It is necessary for growth and healthy hair, skin and nails. Great sources include spinach, broccoli, asparagus, almonds and collard greens.

B3 (Niacin) – Like B1 and B2, vitamin B3 is essential for the conversion of carbohydrates, fats and protein into usable energy. It also stabilizes blood sugar levels and lowers bad cholesterol levels (LDL). Asparagus, bell peppers, broccoli and Swiss chard contain vitamin B3.

B5 (Pantothenic Acid) – Vitamin B5 is widely known to improve how the body responds to stress and anxiety, by supporting the adrenal glands which release stress hormones. It helps to alleviate conditions such as hair loss, allergies and skin conditions. Excellent sources of this important vitamin include cauliflower, grapefruit, bell peppers, broccoli and asparagus.

B6 (Pyridoxine) – Sometimes referred to as the mood vitamin, B6 is responsible for the production of an important neurotransmitter (brain chemical) called serotonin. Serotonin plays an important role in the regulation of sleep and moods so deficient levels may therefore affect our moods, causing us to feel down in the dumps. Spinach, bell peppers, tomatoes, bananas, kale and broccoli are excellent sources.

Biotin – Belonging to the B vitamin group, biotin is involved in the metabolism of sugar and fat, which is needed for healthy skin and hair, the balancing of blood sugar levels and energy production. Hair loss, muscle cramps and skin conditions such as dermatitis benefit from healthy levels of biotin. Excellent sources include Swiss chard, cucumber, carrots, strawberries and raspberries.

Vitamin B9 (Folic Acid/Folacin/Folate) – Folic acid is required for healthy cell division and reproduction, is important for the formation of red blood cells, supports the nervous system by allowing nerves to function properly and can help to alleviate mental fatigue and irritability. Beets, collard greens, spinach, strawberries, broccoli and papaya contain excellent sources of vitamin B9.

Vitamin B12 (Cobalamin) – Vitamin B12 helps to metabolize protein, fats and carbohydrates for usable energy. It is also essential for the development of nerve cells and the formation of red blood cells. Symptoms associated with B12 deficiency include dandruff, fatigue, menstrual problems and paleness. Salmon and sardines are excellent sources of vitamin B12.

Vitamin C

Vitamin C is an all rounder vitamin as far as I am concerned, possessing numerous health benefits. An important point to take into consideration is the fact that it is a water soluble vitamin and therefore cannot be stored in the body. As a result, foods rich in this important vitamin must be consumed on a daily basis to replenish depleted levels. It is essential for the formation of collagen and important for the health of our bones, teeth and cartilage. It improves iron absorption preventing anaemia, lowers bad cholesterol (LDL), is essential for the proper function of the human eye and is a powerful antioxidant, protecting the cells from free radical damage. Sources of vitamin C are best consumed raw as it is easily destroyed during the cooking process. Oranges, lemons, cauliflower, parsley, broccoli, strawberries, bell peppers and kale are rich supplies.

Vitamin D

Vitamin D is essential for the regulation of bone and muscle health by enabling the body to properly absorb and use calcium, the mineral required for healthy bone development and maintenance. Also known for decreasing high blood pressure, helping to prevent type II diabetes and supporting mood stability, vitamin D is a vital addition to a healthy diet. The best and most natural source of vitamin D is sunlight. Dietary sources include milk, eggs, liver and oily fish such as mackerel and sardines.

Vitamin E

A powerful antioxidant, vitamin E helps to prevent cell damage from free radicals. It is an excellent healer of the skin, repairing and strengthening cells. It also protects from the harmful effects of the sun's UV rays. It is plentiful is dandelion greens, spinach, collards, avocado, chard, almonds, asparagus and bell peppers.

Vitamin K

This is a fat soluble vitamin and is extremely important in the process of blood clot formation, allowing the blood to clot normally. Recommended doses of vitamin K ensures healthy bones by preventing fractures, it also helps to prevent calcification of arteries. It is found in abundance in green beans, spinach, Swiss chard, broccoli, kale, brussel sprouts, celery, cabbage, carrots, tomatoes and blueberries.

M inerals are the keystones to our health, they are critical for the proper functioning of the body. Because minerals are not produced by our bodies, it is essential we obtain them from the food we consume on a daily basis. There are over 100 minerals but the ones necessary for good health are detailed below;

Boron

Boron is an essential trace mineral, used to maintain the health of bones and is widely used in the treatment of arthritis. It also plays a vital role in sexual health, muscle pain and brain function. One of the best dietary sources of boron includes apples. Pears, oranges, grapes and kiwi fruit also contain this important mineral.

Calcium

Well known for maintaining the strength of our bones and teeth, calcium also plays a significant role in other areas of our health including reducing the risk of heart disease, weight loss, menopause and reducing the symptoms of PMS. Spinach, kale, cabbage and sesame seeds are excellent sources.

Chromium

Chromium is an important mineral in that it monitors our blood sugar levels and helps to stabilize blood sugar levels by regulating insulin production in the body. It also helps with weight loss by reducing the feeling of hunger, acts as a good friend to our cardiovascular system helping to reduce the risk of heart disease and prevents high blood pressure. Dietary sources include peas, onions, brewer's yeast and tomatoes.

Copper

Found in asparagus, kale, spinach, Swiss chard and sesame seeds, copper helps to maintain our energy levels though iron absorption. It also helps to keep our immune system strong and maintains the health of bones and connective tissues.

Iodine

Iodine is vital for the healthy functioning of the thyroid gland which in turn has an important influence on the metabolic processes in the body. In other words, it helps to utilize calories, preventing their storage as excess fats. Excellent sources include salmon, sea bass, spinach, sesame seeds, Swiss chard and garlic.

Iron

Iron is responsible for helping the blood carry oxygen around the body thereby keeping our immune systems strong and keeping you feeling energized. Symptoms of an iron deficiency include feeling tired and weak, decreased focus and dizziness. Dark green vegetables are excellent sources of iron including spinach, Swiss chard, asparagus, collard greens, romaine lettuce and cabbage.

Magnesium

Magnesium helps to maintain the normal functioning of the nervous system. It also helps to work the muscles and strengthens bones. Headaches, muscle weakness and imbalanced sugar levels are common symptoms of a body low in magnesium. Swiss chard, spinach and collard greens are excellent sources.

Phosphorus

Primarily regarded for its role in bone health, phosphorus has other important functions too. It is effective in relieving digestive disorders such as diarrhoea and constipation, improving mental clarity, maintaining proper cell reproduction and producing and regulating hormones. Excellent sources include sardines, pumpkin seeds, sesame seeds and flax seeds.

Antioxidants come in a variety of different forms so it is important you have an understanding of what they are and how they benefit our health, as almost all fruit and vegetables contain various levels of this important nutrient.

Antioxidants are powerful nutrients that can slow oxidative damage to our body's tissues, preventing free radical damage. "Free Radicals" is a term you will hear quite often when it comes to our health. These bad boys are either produced by the cells in our body or are introduced from our outside environment, for example, exhaust fumes. They are unstable molecules that are missing an electron, and in order to become more stable they attack and destroy other healthy molecules to get the missing electron they need. This creates a domino type effect amongst the cells in our body as one attacks the other.

The job of antioxidants is to neutralize these free radicals. However, if the body does not have an adequate supply of antioxidants, it will be overcome with free radicals which eventually cause early aging of the skin, illness and in some cases, cancer legions.

Can you imagine the damage an unhealthy diet causes to our bodies over a long period of time? Eating foods rich in antioxidants is therefore vitally important.

CHAPTER THREE
Smoothie Ingredients – Health Benefits

F ruit is one of nature's most magnificent creations, packed with numerous vitamins, minerals, phytonutrients, dietary fibre and antioxidants. It comes in all shapes and sizes, in all colours of the rainbow and tastes absolutely delicious.

Fruit's resume of health benefits could quite easily fill this entire book but for now I will try and condense them into just one chapter;

* Protecting and rejuvenating tissues and cells
* Prolonging or reversing the signs of aging
* Rejuvenating organs
* Healthy eyes
* Lustrous hair
* Strong nails
* Rock solid immune system
* Preventing osteoporosis
* Lowering of blood pressure
* Caner fighting properties

As you can see, incorporating fruit in your smoothies is a fantastic way to include this food phenomenon into your diet.

Apples
"An apple a day keeps the doctor away". An old adage which happens to be very true. Apples are particularly notorious for their impressive list of phytonutrients and antioxidants, flavonoids – catechin and quercetin, are powerful examples. Research has shown that these compounds have been known to protect the body from the effects of free radicals thereby reducing the risk of various cancers. Apples also

contain a valuable source of soluble fibre known as pectin which can have the effect of lowering bad cholesterol (known as LDL) and regulating blood sugar. Vitamin C, beta carotene, riboflavin, thiamin, potassium, phosphorus and calcium are also found in this super fruit.

Acai Berry

Acai extracts have been used to treat digestive disorders by the Amazon Basin tribes for many years. Their dietary fibre content together with the linoleic acid and oleic acid (omega 6 & 9) found in these berries, means that they reduce bad cholesterol (LDL), thus preventing heart disease. They also contain anti-aging and anti-inflammatory properties making them an ideal ingredient for detox smoothies. B complex vitamins, vitamin K, iron, copper, potassium and magnesium are further essential nutrients found in acai berries, all helping to promote health and well being.

Apricots

Apricots might be small but they are jam-packed full of essential nutrients. These beautiful orange coloured fruits have a high beta carotene content making them an important prevention against heart disease, while also reducing bad cholesterol. They are excellent sources of vitamins A & C, which are powerful antioxidants. Apricots are also a rich source of fibre, a nutrient vital for a successful weight loss plan. Healthy high fibre foods make you feel full, eliminating the need to snack.

Avocados

Some people may be a little wary of avocados especially due to their high fat content. But what you need to be aware of is that the fat found in avocados is largely monounsaturated fat which is actually very beneficial to our health, helping to lower bad cholesterol. Avocados also contain an amazing array of phytonutrients, vitamin C, vitamins B5 & B6, vitamin K, potassium and dietary fibre.

Bananas

Whether eaten sliced over a cereal, mashed up on healthy brown bread or blended in a smoothie, bananas are a delicious healthy snack loved by adults and children alike. 3 very important facts to know about bananas are that they are relatively low in calories (about 100 calories per 1 medium banana); they are high in fibre and contain even higher amounts of potassium. Dietary fibre not only helps lower the risk of developing heart disease but it also enhances weight loss while potassium plays a vital role in maintaining proper fluid balance in the body. Vitamin B6 is also found in abundance in bananas and is essential in cell formation and normal nervous system function.

Blackberries

Blackberries are one of the highest fibre fruits in the world. They can be eaten fresh or frozen and are a fantastically nutritious ingredient in a smoothie. Rich in vitamins, minerals and antioxidants, blackberries not only pack a powerful nutritious punch but they are also low in calories. Just some of the benefits of eating this delicious fruit include anti aging, a reduction in the risk of cancer, a reduction in the risk of heart disease, improvement in brain function and better circulation.

Blueberries

Blueberries have superstar status when it comes to their health benefits. Highly regarded as having the highest level of antioxidants among all fruits and vegetables, they truly are a nutrient powerhouse. Polyphenols, powerful antioxidants found in blueberries, have been attributed to helping virtually all diseases and disorders. They neutralize free radicals, preventing damage to our cell structures and DNA, resulting in a strong immune system, strong connective tissue, improvement in collagen structures and a healthy heart. Blueberries also contain vitamin C, B complex vitamins, vitamin A, vitamin E, iron, zinc and selenium.

Cherries

Sweet or sour, cherries are bursting with nutrients. They are loaded with anti aging, anti inflammatory and cancer fighting agents. Studies have shown that a diet high in cherries helps to reduce the risk of cancer, heart disease, high blood pressure, obesity, bad cholesterol and inflammation. Along with their superior antioxidant supply, they are also a good source of vitamins and minerals including vitamin C, vitamin A, potassium, zinc, copper and iron.

Cranberries

Cranberries are widely known for their successful treatment of urinary tract infections. However, they have an array of other health benefits which should not be overlooked. Containing some of the most potent antioxidants of any fruit, research indicates that cranberries may protect against cancer and heart disease, may reduce inflammation and prevent the formation of kidney stones. Vitamin C, vitamin E, vitamin K, dietary fibre, potassium and phosphorus are also found in this magical fruit.

Clementines

These small, sweetly flavoured citrus fruits are not only very tasty but have numerous health benefits. They have a rich antioxidant supply which protects the body from negative effects of free radicals. The high vitamin C, beta carotene and fibre content, means that clementines help with the treatment of digestive disorders, collagen production and poor vision.

Grapes

Widely popular, grapes have a wealth of antioxidant nutrients ranging from vitamin C and beta carotene to manganese and resveratrol. Resveratrol is a powerful compound with numerous health benefits including, protection against prostate and colon cancers, heart disease and the treatment of Alzheimer's disease. Grapes are also rich sources of vitamin A, potassium, phosphorus and calcium.

Grapefruit

Grapefruits contain the magical anti inflammatory and skin cleansing enzyme, bromelain, making them a perfect choice food for a weight loss plan. Many dieticians recommend eating only grapefruits or drinking fresh grapefruit juice for 3 days to eliminate cellulite. They are loaded with vitamins A and C while also being good sources of vitamins B1 and B5. The antioxidant, lycopene, is found in abundance in red and pink grapefruits which is known to be most effective in helping to fight free radicals which can damage our cell structures.

Kiwi

In my opinion the benefits of kiwi fruit have been massively overlooked. These wonderful little exotic fruits are decidedly one of the richest sources of nutrients for our body. They contain the highest content of vitamin C, almost twice as much as an orange. Not only that but kiwi's are also jam packed with antioxidants, have a high dietary fibre content and contain excellent levels of vitamin E and potassium. The health benefits of this superstar fruit include anti-aging, anti-inflammatory, cancer fighting, protection from free radical damage, controlling blood sugar levels and protection against asthma.

Lemons

Lemons have been used over the years for detoxification of the body, helping to cleanse the liver. As a result, weight loss is accelerated, our skin becomes clearer, our digestive system becomes more efficient and our energy increases. Lemons also contain unique flavonoid compounds resulting in excellent anti-cancer and anti-inflammatory properties. Vitamin C is also found in abundance in this nutritious fruit.

Lime

The smallest of the citrus fruits, limes became famous for their successful treatment of scurvy, a disease caused by the deficiency of vitamin C. Symptoms include flu, cough, cracked lips, mouth ulcers and bleeding gums. Loaded with the powerful antioxidant vitamin C, limes strengthen the immune system and fights against free radical damage, keeping our bodies healthy and strong.

Mangos

Besides being deliciously sweet and irresistible, mangos are very nutritionally rich fruits, containing an assortment of health benefits. Their high vitamin A and beta carotene content makes them an ideal tonic for our skin as the antioxidants fight free radical damage of the cells. Mangos are also an excellent source of fibre which is an important nutrient for a healthy heart and digestive system. Vitamins C, B6, E, potassium and magnesium are also present in this wondrous fruit.

Nectarines

Nectarines are similar to peaches or plums and have a juicy unique taste. They are a great snack when on a weight loss plan as one medium sized nectarine contains approximately 60 calories and is fat free. Packed with antioxidants, this mouth watering fruit helps your body fight off cancer as well as other diseases. Nectarines are also a great source of fibre and potassium.

Oranges

Oranges are one of the world's most popular fruits, and are renowned for their concentration of vitamin C. Their list of other essential vitamins and minerals makes for an impressive read. They contain an array of phytochemicals and flavonoids which contain important anti-cancer, anti-inflammatory and anti-aging properties. Oranges also contain high levels of fibre and calcium, the fibre being fantastic at balancing our blood sugar levels, and the calcium at maintaining healthy bones and teeth.

Peaches
While peaches are not included on the super fruits list, they still contain enough levels of essential vitamins and minerals to be considered as healthy nutritious snacks. Carotene, found in peaches, is converted to vitamin A when ingested. This powerful antioxidant helps to maintain a healthy heart while also maintaining our vision. Vitamin B3 (Niacin) is also found in this juicy delight, playing an important role in our bodies' energy metabolism.

Pears
These juicy beauties are not only sweet and delicious but offer a wealth of health benefiting nutrients, including a large amount of dietary fibre, vitamin C, vitamin K, vitamins B2 and B3, calcium, copper and potassium. At approximately 100 calories per medium pear, health care practitioners often recommend including pears as part of a sensible diet plan.

Pineapples
Pineapples are just balls of tropical, lush sweetness, making them one of the most cherished fruits on the planet. Even better still, they are really good for you! The 2 most notable ingredients found in pineapples include bromelain and manganese. Bromelain, a rich source of enzymes, is excellent for digestion as it helps the body digest proteins more efficiently. Manganese is an essential trace mineral needed for strong bones, healthy skin and strong connective tissue. The high vitamin C content also adds to this fruit's super powers.

Pomegranate
These beautiful reddish-pink coloured fruits have become very popular over recent times as more studies have shown that pomegranates contain a rich supply of phytochemicals, antioxidant

powerhouses that are wonderful heart and skin tonics. Pomegranate juice, known to be more concentrated, is considered a health elixir, fighting against many cancers, Alzheimer's and high blood pressure.

Raspberry

It is hard to know which berry is more nutritious but raspberries are definitely high on the list. The variety of anti-inflammatory and antioxidant properties in this fruit is second to none, protecting us from free radical damage, obesity and many more diseases and disorders. Raspberries also provide bountiful levels of fibre, with one cup containing a massive 8 grams. Vitamin C, vitamin K, potassium, copper and manganese are also found in these delicious berries.

Strawberry

Nutrient rich and packed with antioxidants, strawberries are one of the healthiest fruits to include in your diet. With high levels of vitamin C, folate, dietary fibre, potassium, manganese, omega 3 fatty acids and vitamin K, it is no wonder they are on the top 10 superfood's list of almost every nutritional book and website in the world.

Watermelon

If you are not already a fan of watermelon then please go to your nearest fruit market and by lots of it! We really don't hear enough about this gloriously healthy fruit. Did you know that watermelon contains the highest concentration of lycopene of any fresh fruit or vegetable on the market? Lycopene is a powerful antioxidant that neutralizes free radicals in the body and has fantastic cancer fighting properties. Extremely high in water (approximately 95%), watermelons have become a popular food choice for dieters due to their filling effect. They are also rich in vitamin A, vitamin C, potassium and magnesium.

V egetables play an important role in everyone's diet, containing dozens of vital nutrients to keep the body strong and healthy. With a variety of different types, the nutritional content of vegetables can vary greatly. Leafy greens such as romaine lettuce or arugula for example, are considered to be the most concentrated sources of antioxidants, essential vitamins and minerals and dietary fibre.

Leafy greens are the most popular vegetable of choice for healthy smoothie making. There is very little preparation time with them and they blend well with almost all fruits.

Another important variety of vegetable includes Cruciferous vegetables, belonging to the Brassicaceae family. Examples include, broccoli, kale, cabbage and watercress. Really packing a nutritional punch, they contain large amounts of dietary fibre, multiple phytochemicals and vital vitamins and minerals.

Root vegetables are another variety that must also be considered. For the purposes of this book, the most common examples include beet, carrots and celery. All 3 contain fabulous detoxification properties, perfect for weight loss smoothies.

Most vegetables are available all year round but tend to be best picked during the winter months. Always try and choose organic so to avoid any pesticides or artificial chemicals. Fresh is best, look for firm vegetables, not overripe or damaged. Always wash your produce thoroughly before consuming.

Arugula
This delicate, leafy green salad vegetable, also known as rocket, might be small in size but is large when it comes to its nutritional content. Arugula contains large amounts of vitamin K and calcium, both essential for healthy bones and teeth. It is a popular choice among dieters as it contains high levels of chlorophyll, an important

substance for detoxifying the liver. Fibre, folate, vitamin B, antioxidants and phytochemicals are also found in this flavoursome leaf.

Asparagus
Synonymous with the beginning of spring, asparagus is low in calories and high in nutrients. It contains a whopping amount of potassium and fibre, both excellent for the proper functioning of the digestive system. Vitamins A, B & K, folate and a healthy dose of flavonoids are also found in this herbaceous plant. Eating asparagus may help to protect against certain forms of cancer due to its high glutathione content, a detoxifying compound.

Beets
Fight cancer, reverse the signs of aging and ensure healthy cell production with this nutritious and delicious root vegetable. Beets purify our blood making them a wonderful tonic for the liver. They contain vitamins A & C, magnesium, potassium, iron, beta carotene, folic acid and fibre. While the root is uber nutritious, don't forget the leaves, as their nutritional value is even higher, especially in vitamins A & C.

Bok Choy
This nutrient dense food is a type of Chinese cabbage that contains protein, fibre and almost all the essential vitamins and minerals a body needs to stay healthy. Some of the main reasons we should include bok choy in our diet include, its ability to protect our cells from free radical damage due to the high vitamins A & C content, its ability to build and maintain strong bones due to the calcium, vitamin K and potassium content and its ability to maintain cognitive function due to the folic acid content. It tastes really good too!

Broccoli

Love it or hate it, you cannot help but be in awe of the King of the Cruciferous vegetables. Broccoli is a nutritional wonder food, containing so many essential vitamins and minerals. It provides a highly concentrated source of vitamin C, high levels of calcium and vitamin K, a high amount of potassium, magnesium and calcium, a healthy dose of fibre and too many disease-fighting antioxidants to mention. The perfect all rounder!

Cabbage

Another significant member of the Cruciferous family, cabbage comes in a variety of colours, shapes and sizes. It also contains an array of nutrients, including an abundance of vitamin C, fibre, beta carotene, vitamin K, calcium, iodine and magnesium. Purple cabbage contains important flavonoids called anthocyanins, powerful antioxidants that protect our body from toxic damage. In conclusion, adding cabbage to a well balanced diet could help you live a long healthy life.

Celery

Popular among dieters for its amazing detoxification properties, celery also has many other health benefits that should not be ignored. Phthalides found in celery help to relax the muscles of arteries thereby regulating blood pressure, its natural sodium content balances the pH of the blood, neutralizing acidity and it contains vital antioxidants that have cancer fighting and immune boosting properties.

Chard (Swiss)

When you think of highly nutritious green vegetables, it astounds me the number of people who do not even consider Swiss chard. Big mistake people! Swiss chard is one of the most antioxidant rich foods on the planet, containing ample amounts of vitamins A, C & E, beta carotene, lutein, zeaxanthin, betalaine, zinc and many more. It also provides a rich mineral supply, along with tons of dietary fibre.

Carrots

This crunchy sweet vegetable not only tastes delicious but is also jam packed with vitamins B & C, beta carotene, potassium, phosphorus and dietary fibre. Remember when your Mom used to say that if you eat more carrots you would be able to see in the dark?! Well, while this may not be entirely true (eh...hem Mom), carrots do contain vitamin A and zeaxanthin, important antioxidants that help protect the eyes against cataracts and improve night blindness.

Collard Greens

Collard greens are gaining popularity in the world of healthy eating, and for good reason. They are loaded with vitamin A, mostly in the form of beta carotene, which has been shown to contain cancer fighting and anti aging properties. They are also highly regarded for their vitamin C and fibre content, are low in calories and help to maintain a healthy immune system.

> **Chlorophyll:** *is a substance found in plants, a green pigment enabling plants to absorb light from the sun and then convert this light into usable energy (photosynthesis). It also supplies our bodies with many vital antioxidants and powerful anti-carcinogenic properties, found in abundance in kale, Swiss chard, collard greens, spinach, romaine lettuce and broccoli.*

Dandelion

Regarded by some people as a pesky weed that grows in the garden, dandelion has actually gained a distinguished reputation as a medicinal miracle plant, used for detoxification purposes around the world. It would take another book to list all the health benefits of dandelion but probably the most significant is the profound effect it has on the liver. Liver detoxification is absolutely vital for the human body to remain in a healthy state and dandelion ranks as the number one choice to help with this.

Kale

You may have seen the term ORAC mentioned a few times in various nutrition books and articles. It stands for Oxygen Radical Absorbance Capacity and is basically used to measure the level of antioxidants present in a particular food. Simply put, the higher the ORAC value, the more antioxidants that food will have, meaning it will have more disease fighting capabilities. Guess what vegetable has the highest ORAC ranking? Kale. And it doesn't stop there. Not only is this delicious vegetable an antioxidant superhero but it also contains a rich supply of vitamins A, C and K, calcium, iron, omega 3 fatty acids and essential dietary fibre.

Peppers (Sweet)

Bell peppers come in a variety of beautiful colours and shapes and are an excellent way to brighten up otherwise bland dishes. While all peppers are good for you, red peppers are the most potent when it comes to their antioxidant content. They contain a rich supply of vitamins A, C and K, fibre, B vitamins, iron, copper and selenium, contributing to a healthy liver, healthy skin and a strong immune system.

Romaine Lettuce

The nutritional content of romaine lettuce is surprising to many people and provides for an interesting read. One head of this nutritious leafy green contains rich supplies of calcium, vitamin C (more than an orange), iron, beta carotene, protein and copper. Because of its high water and low calorie content it is a popular choice for many dieters and works wonders in any salad or smoothie.

Spinach

Second to kale on the ORAC scale, spinach is one of the richest sources of essential nutrients on the planet. It provides the body with high levels of fibre, vitamins C and E, beta carotene and selenium. These in turn give us a clear healthy complexion, strong connective tissue, brighter eyes, a rock solid immune system and more energy. Popeye was right!

Tomatoes

Many a debate has been had about whether a tomato is a fruit or vegetable. To answer the $64,000 question, technically it's a fruit as it is developed in the base of a flower but seriously, who cares?! Fruit or vegetable, it doesn't alter the fact that these beautiful red treats are packed full of important vitamins such as vitamins A, C and E. What makes them stand out from the crowd is their lycopene content. Lycopene is a powerful antioxidant associated with significant cancer fighting capabilities such as prostate cancer in men, lung, stomach and cervical cancers. In my book that makes it an important addition to any diet!

Watercress

This pungent delicate herb has slowly crept up on the list of top superfoods. Not only is it practically calorie free but it contains just as much vitamin C as oranges, just as much iron as spinach and just as much vitamin A as celery. Its health benefits range from a strong immune system to a healthy heart.

CHAPTER FOUR
Smoothie Bases & Boosters

Healthy smoothies are not just about their fruit and vegetable content. A smoothie needs a healthy base before it can be classed as nutritious, it is the foundation of all your smoothies. There is no point adding tons of vitamin laden fruits to your recipe, only to add a fruit juice with artificial colours and flavourings or a teaspoon of sugar.

The good news is there are plenty of healthy choices on the market today, ones that will give you a nutritional boost without adding extra calories to your diet. Always remember, the base can be just as important as the ingredients!

We will now take a more detailed look at the various bases and boosters that can make our smoothies even more delicious and nutritious.

Bases
Before I list the healthiest bases to use, I want to start by giving you 3 bases that I do not recommend using:

1. **Sugar laden fruit juice** – most fruit juices sold in supermarkets contain massive amounts of sugar and can add an extra couple of hundred calories to your smoothie, always read the label before buying. Always go for unsweetened fruit juices or better still, juice your own.

2. **Ordinary tap water** – while some tap water may be ok, studies have shown that it may contain trace amounts of harmful substances such as lead, perchlorate, fluoride and chlorine.

3. Regular milk – cows being over milked, fed hormones and other various chemicals unfortunately means that supermarket milk may not be as healthy as once considered.

Switch from the above and try any of the following:

Almond milk – always choose plain almond milk with no added sugar. A healthy alternative to normal milk, it contains rich doses of vitamins A, B, D & E and a moderate amount of iron.

Soy milk – soy milk, made from soy beans, is high in essential omega 3 & 6 fatty acids, fibre, vitamins and phytoestrogen. Always choose fortified soy milk due to its higher calcium content.

Pomegranate juice – high on the ORAC scale, this wonderful juice is loaded with polyphenols, essential for a toxin free body. Vitamins C & K, potassium and folic acid are also present. I recommend unsweetened and organic.

Cranberry juice – highly effective in the treatment of urinary and bladder infections, this tart tasting juice contains high levels of vitamin C and antioxidants. I recommend unsweetened and organic.

Acai berry juice – the acai berry has one of the highest ORAC values found in plants, making it an antioxidant powerhouse. It also contains vitamins C & E, fibre and essential fatty acids.

Noni juice – growing in popularity, noni juice contains a good source of vitamin C along with strong antioxidant properties.

Green tea – used for centuries by Chinese people, green tea is rich in catechin polyphenols, a powerful antioxidant with plentiful cancer fighting and health promoting properties. It has also been known to aid weight loss and prevent tooth decay.

Chamomile tea – widely known for its sleep inducing properties, chamomile tea has many other health benefits such as relieving stomach cramps, irritable bowel syndrome and skin conditions such as eczema and psoriasis.

Coconut water – popular among celebs and athletes, coconut water is rich in natural electrolytes, minerals needed by the body for normal functioning. The most important, potassium, is essential for maintaining water balance in the body.

Wheatgrass juice – a miracle juice extracted from the blades of wheatgrass. Nutrient dense, it contains a large spectrum of antioxidants, phytochemicals and vitamins.

Boosters

Adding boosters to a smoothie is a fantastic way to considerably enhance its nutritional content. Thankfully, there are plenty of nutrient dense boosters that are quick and easy to use and can be added to any smoothie recipe.

Bee pollen – this nutrient dense superfood extracted from the nectar of flowers, contains all 8 essential amino acids, protein, dozens of vitamins and minerals and healthy enzymes, all required to maintain a healthy body.

Spirulina – a blue-green algae, Spirulina is often deemed the most nutritionally dense superfood on the market. It contains high levels of chlorophyll, vitamins A and B, protein, iron and is an extremely rich source of beta carotene.

Protein powder – protein powder is essential for the growth and maintenance of muscles and maintaining healthy bones. When choosing your brand, make sure it is low fat, contains low amounts of sugary carbohydrates and has a high serving of good protein. Your body needs 1g of protein for every 1kg of body weight.

Coconut oil – derived from the meat of coconuts, this amazing superfood contains essential fatty acids, is rich in antioxidants and has important anti-bacterial agents.

Flax seed – whether it's the oil or seeds, flax seeds are a rich source of omega 3 fatty acids. The seeds are a great source of fibre, antioxidants and magnesium with an array of health benefits ranging from healthy skin to lower cholesterol.

Hemp seed – hemp seeds are a fantastic source of protein and contain all essential amino acids. They are also rich in omega 3 and 6 oil, phytochemicals and important antioxidants.

Manuka honey – different to normal honey, manuka honey has many anti-bacterial, anti-fungal and anti-inflammatory properties. It has a UMF which stands for Unique Manuka Factor, the higher the UMF, the higher the anti-bacterial properties it contains. I always go for a UMF of 10+ or more.

Sprouts – there are many types of sprouts to choose from, all healthy in their own right. Examples include broccoli, soybean and radish. They are rich in good protein and contain many essential vitamins and minerals including vitamins A, C, E, K, potassium, magnesium and many others.

Matcha green tea powder – when you drink matcha powder you are ingesting the whole leaf and not just the brewed tea, making the powder much more nutrient dense. Green tea contains cancer fighting, anti-aging and anti-inflammatory properties.

CHAPTER FIVE
Smoothie Ingredients – Nutritional Content

Fruit	Nutritional Value	How to Prepare
Apple **182g** **One medium apple, raw with skin.** Calories - 95 Protein - 0.5g Fibre - 4.4g	Vit A - 98.28IU Vit B1 (thiamin) - 0.031mg Vit B2 (Riboflavin) - 0.047mg Vit B3 (Niacin) - 0.166mg Vit B6 - 0.075mg Vit C - 8.37mg Folate - 5.46µg Vit E - 0.33mg Vit K - 4µg Potassium - 194.74mg Calcium - 10.92mg Phosphorus - 20.02mg Magnesium - 9.1mg	Wash thoroughly. Core apple and make sure to remove all seeds before blending.
Avocado **201g** **One fruit.** Calories - 322 Protein - 4g Fibre - 13.5g	Vit A - 293.46IU Vit B1 (thiamin) - 0.135mg Vit B2 (Riboflavin) - 0.261mg Vit B3 (Niacin) - 3.493mg Vit B6 - 0.517mg Vit C - 20.1mg Folate - 162.81µg Vit E - 4.16mg Vit K - 42.21µg Potassium - 974.85mg Calcium - 24.12mg Phosphorus - 104.52mg Magnesium - 58.29mg	Cut in half to remove pit and chop.

Fruit	Nutritional Value	How to Prepare
Banana **118g** **One medium sized banana.** Calories - 105 Protein - 1.3g Fibre - 3.1g	Vit A - 75.52IU Vit B1 (thiamin) - 0.037mg Vit B2 (Riboflavin) - 0.086mg Vit B3 (Niacin) - 0.785mg Vit B6 - 0.433mg Vit C - 10.27mg Folate - 23.6µg Vit E - 0.12mg Vit K - 0.59µg Potassium - 422.44mg Calcium - 5.9mg Phosphorus - 25.96mg Magnesium - 31.86mg	Peel and slice.
Blackberries **144g** **One cup of blackberries.** Calories - 62 Protein - 2g Fibre - 7.6g	Vit A - 308IU Vit B1 (thiamin) - 0.029mg Vit B2 (Riboflavin) - 0.037mg Vit B3 (Niacin) - 0.93mg Vit B6 - 0.043mg Vit C - 30.2mg Folate - 36µg Vit E - 1.68mg Vit K - 28.5µg Potassium - 233mg Calcium - 41.76mg Phosphorus - 31.68mg Magnesium - 28.8mg	Wash thoroughly in a strainer.

Fruit	Nutritional Value	How to Prepare
Blackcurrants **112g** **One cup of Blackcurrants.** Calories - 71 Protein - 1.6g Fibre - 4g	Vit A - 258IU Vit B1 (thiamin) - 0.056mg Vit B2 (Riboflavin) - 0.056mg Vit B3 (Niacin) - 0.336mg Vit B6 - 0.074mg Vit C - 202.7mg Vit E - 1.12mg Potassium - 361mg Calcium - 62mg Phosphorus - 66mg Magnesium - 27mg	Wash thoroughly in a strainer.
Blueberries **148g** **One cup of blueberries.** Calories - 84 Protein - 1.1g Fibre - 3.6g	Vit A - 79.92IU Vit B1 (thiamin) - 0.055mg Vit B2 (Riboflavin) - 0.061mg Vit B3 (Niacin) - 0.619mg Vit B6 - 0.077mg Vit C - 14.36mg Folate - 8.88µg Vit E - 0.84mg Vit K - 28.56µg Potassium - 113.96mg Calcium - 8.88mg Phosphorus - 17.76mg Magnesium - 8.88mg	Wash thoroughly in a strainer.

Fruit	Nutritional Value	How to Prepare
Cherries 154g **One cup of sweet, raw cherries without pits.** Calories - 97 Protein - 1.6g Fibre - 3.2g	Vit A - 98.56IU Vit B1 (thiamin) - 0.042mg Vit B2 (Riboflavin) - 0.051mg Vit B3 (Niacin) - 0.237mg Vit B6 - 0.075mg Vit C - 10.78mg Folate - 6.16µg Vit E - 0.11mg Vit K - 3.23µg Potassium - 341.88mg Calcium - 20.02mg Phosphorus - 32.34mg Magnesium - 16.94mg	Remove the stalks and wash thoroughly in a strainer. Remove the pits in the centre of the fruit before blending.
Cranberries 100g **One cup of raw whole cranberries.** Calories - 46 Protein - 0.4g Fibre - 4.6g	Vit A - 60IU Vit B1 (thiamin) - 0.012mg Vit B2 (Riboflavin) - 0.02mg Vit B3 (Niacin) - 0.101mg Vit B6 - 0.057mg Vit C - 13.3mg Folate - 1µg Vit E - 1.2mg Vit K - 5.1µg Potassium - 85mg Calcium - 8mg Phosphorus - 13mg Magnesium - 6mg	Rinse the fruit in a strainer immediately before blending.

Fruit	Nutritional Value	How to Prepare
Grapefruit 256g **One medium sized pink, red, or white grapefruit.** Calories - 82 Protein - 1.6g Fibre - 2.8g	Vit A - 2373.12IU Vit B1 (thiamin) - 0.092mg Vit B2 (Riboflavin) - 0.052mg Vit B3 (Niacin) - 0.64mg Vit B6 - 0.108mg Vit C - 88.06mg Folate - 25.6µg Vit E - 0.34mg Vit K - 0.0µg Potassium - 355.84mg Calcium - 30.72mg Phosphorus - 20.48mg Magnesium - 20.48mg	Peel off the skin thinly, keeping as much of the white pith on as possible (this contains the highest amount of essential bioflavonoids and cancer fighting properties). Cut into segments to fit into the blender.
Grapes 151g **One cup of raw, red or green seedless grapes.** Calories - 104 Protein - 1.1g Fibre - 1.4g	Vit A - 99.66IU Vit B1 (thiamin) - 0.104mg Vit B2 (Riboflavin) - 0.106mg Vit B3 (Niacin) - 0.284mg Vit B6 - 0.13mg Vit C - 4.83mg Folate - 3.02µg Vit E - 0.29mg Vit K - 22.05µg Potassium - 288.41mg Calcium - 15.1mg Phosphorus - 30.2mg Magnesium - 10.57mg	Remove grapes from stems and wash thoroughly.

Fruit	Nutritional Value	How to Prepare
Kiwi Fruit **69g** **One kiwi fruit, 2"** **diameter.** Calories - 42 Protein - 0.8g Fibre - 2.1g	Vit A - 60.03IU Vit B1 (thiamin) - 0.019mg Vit B2 (Riboflavin) - 0.017mg Vit B3 (Niacin) - 0.235mg Vit B6 - 0.043mg Vit C - 63.96mg Folate - 17.25µg Vit E - 1.01mg Vit K - 27.81µg Potassium - 215.28mg Calcium - 23.46mg Phosphorus - 23.46mg Magnesium - 11.73mg	Peel the fruit and chop into 6 pieces.
Lemon **7g** **One wedge of lemon,** **raw without peel.** Calories - 2 Protein - 0.1g Fibre - 0.2g	Vit A - 1.54IU Vit B1 (thiamin) - 0.003mg Vit B2 (Riboflavin) - 0.001mg Vit B3 (Niacin) - 0.007mg Vit B6 - 0.006mg Vit C - 3.71mg Folate - 0.77µg Vit E - 0.01mg Vit K - 0.0µg Potassium - 9.66mg Calcium - 1.82mg Phosphorus - 1.12mg Magnesium - 0.56mg	Peel off the skin thinly, keeping as much of the white pith on as possible (this contains the highest amount of essential bioflavonoids and cancer fighting properties). Cut into segments to fit into the juicer.

Fruit	Nutritional Value	How to Prepare
Lime **67g** **One whole lime.** Calories - 20 Protein - 0.5g Fibre - 1.9g	Vit A - 33.5IU Vit B1 (thiamin) - 0.02mg Vit B2 (Riboflavin) - 0.013mg Vit B3 (Niacin) - 0.134mg Vit B6 - 0.029mg Vit C - 19.5mg Folate - 5.36µg Vit E - 0.15mg Vit K - 0.4µg Potassium - 68.34mg Calcium - 22.11mg Phosphorus - 12.06mg Magnesium - 4.02mg	Peel off the skin thinly, keep as much of the white pith on as possible (this contains the highest amount of essential bioflavonoids and cancer fighting properties). Cut into segments to fit into the blender.
Mango **165g** **One cup of mango pieces.** Calories - 99 Protein - 1.4g Fibre - 2.6g	Vit A - 1785.3IU Vit B1 (thiamin) - 0.046mg Vit B2 (Riboflavin) - 0.063mg Vit B3 (Niacin) - 1.104mg Vit B6 - 0.196mg Vit C - 60.06mg Folate - 70.95µg Vit E - 1.49mg Vit K - 6.93µg Potassium - 277.2mg Calcium - 18.15mg Phosphorus - 23.1mg Magnesium - 16.5mg	Peel the skin from the mango and cut into chunks. Discard the seed in the middle.

Fruit	Nutritional Value	How to Prepare
Melon (cantaloupe) 160g **One cup of cantaloupe melon cubes.** Calories - 54 Protein - 1.3g Fibre - 1.4g	Vit A - 5411.2IU Vit B1 (thiamin) - 0.066mg Vit B2 (Riboflavin) - 0.03mg Vit B3 (Niacin) - 1.174mg Vit B6 - 0.115mg Vit C - 58.72mg Folate - 33.6µg Vit E - 0.08mg Vit K - 4.0µg Potassium - 427.2mg Calcium - 14.4mg Phosphorus - 24mg Magnesium - 19.2mg	Cut the melon into quarters and remove the seeds. Peel off the skin and chop into small pieces.
Nectarine 142g **One medium sized nectarine.** Calories - 62 Protein - 1.5g Fibre - 2.4g	Vit A - 471.44IU Vit B1 (thiamin) - 0.048mg Vit B2 (Riboflavin) - 0.038mg Vit B3 (Niacin) - 1.598mg Vit B6 - 0.036mg Vit C - 7.67mg Folate - 7.1µg Vit E - 1.09mg Vit K - 3.12µg Potassium - 285.42mg Calcium - 8.52mg Phosphorus - 36.92mg Magnesium - 12.78mg	Cut the fruit to remove the pit and cut into chunks.

Fruit	Nutritional Value	How to Prepare
Orange **131g** **One whole medium sized orange without peel.** Calories - 62 Protein - 1.2g Fibre - 3.1g	Vit A - 294.75IU Vit B1 (thiamin) - 0.114mg Vit B2 (Riboflavin) - 0.052mg Vit B3 (Niacin) - 0.369mg Vit B6 - 0.079mg Vit C - 69.69mg Folate - 39.3µg Vit E - 0.24mg Vit K - 0.0µg Potassium - 237.11mg Calcium - 52.4mg Phosphorus - 18.34mg Magnesium - 13.1mg	Peel off the skin thinly, keep as much of the white pith on as possible (this contains the highest amount of essential bioflavonoids and cancer fighting properties). Cut into segments to fit into the blender.
Papaya **157g** **One small sized papaya fruit.** Calories - 68 Protein - 0.7g Fibre - 2.7g	Vit A - 1491.5IU Vit B1 (thiamin) - 0.036mg Vit B2 (Riboflavin) - 0.042mg Vit B3 (Niacin) - 0.56mg Vit B6 - 0.06mg Vit C - 95.61mg Folate - 58.09µg Vit E - 0.47mg Vit K - 4.08µg Potassium - 285.74mg Calcium - 31.4mg Phosphorus - 15.7mg Magnesium - 32.97mg	Peel the fruit. Cut it in half lengthwise and scoop out the seeds. Cut the fruit into small pieces.

Fruit	Nutritional Value	How to Prepare
Passion Fruit **18g** **One fruit without refuse.** Calories - 17 Protein - 0.4g Fibre - 1.9g	Vit A - 228.96IU Vit B1 (thiamin) - 0.0mg Vit B2 (Riboflavin) - 0.023mg Vit B3 (Niacin) - 0.27mg Vit B6 - 0.018mg Vit C - 5.4mg Folate - 2.52µg Vit E - 0.0mg Vit K - 0.13µg Potassium - 62.64mg Calcium - 2.16mg Phosphorus - 12.24mg Magnesium - 5.22mg	Cut in half to remove the inner fruit. Discard the outer skin.
Peach **150g** **One medium sized peach.** Calories - 59 Protein - 1.4g Fibre - 2.3g	Vit A - 489IU Vit B1 (thiamin) - 0.036mg Vit B2 (Riboflavin) - 0.047mg Vit B3 (Niacin) - 1.209mg Vit B6 - 0.038mg Vit C - 9.9mg Folate - 6µg Vit E - 1.10mg Vit K - 3.9µg Potassium - 285mg Calcium - 9mg Phosphorus - 30mg Magnesium - 13.5mg	Rinse and cut in half to remove the pit in the centre.

Fruit	Nutritional Value	How to Prepare
Pear **178g** **One medium sized pear.** Calories - 102 Protein - 0.6g Fibre - 5.5g	Vit A - 44.5IU Vit B1 (thiamin) - 0.021mg Vit B2 (Riboflavin) - 0.046mg Vit B3 (Niacin) - 0.287mg Vit B6 - 0.052mg Vit C - 7.65mg Folate - 12.46µg Vit E - 0.21mg Vit K - 7.83µg Potassium - 206.48mg Calcium - 16.02mg Phosphorus - 21.36mg Magnesium - 12.46mg	Remove the stem and wash the fruit thoroughly. Slice the pear in half and remove the core and seeds.
Pineapple **165g** **One cup of pineapple chunks.** Calories - 82 Protein - 0.9g Fibre - 2.3g	Vit A - 95.71IU Vit B1 (thiamin) - 0.13mg Vit B2 (Riboflavin) - 0.053mg Vit B3 (Niacin) - 0.825mg Vit B6 - 0.185mg Vit C - 78.87mg Folate - 29.7µg Vit E - 0.03mg Vit K - 1.16µg Potassium - 179.85mg Calcium - 21.45mg Phosphorus - 13.2mg Magnesium - 19.8mg	Cut the leaf top off the pineapple and remove the outer layer of skin using a knife. Cut the pineapple into small chunks.

Fruit	Nutritional Value	How to Prepare
Plum **66g** **One fruit.** Calories - 30 Protein - 0.5g Fibre - 0.9g	Vit A - 227.7IU Vit B1 (thiamin) - 0.018mg Vit B2 (Riboflavin) - 0.017mg Vit B3 (Niacin) - 0.275mg Vit B6 - 0.019mg Vit C - 6.27mg Folate - 3.3μg Vit E - 0.17mg Vit K - 4.22μg Potassium - 103.62mg Calcium - 3.96mg Phosphorus - 10.56mg Magnesium - 4.62mg	Wash thoroughly and cut in half to remove the pip.
Raspberries **123g** **One cup of raspberries.** Calories - 64 Protein - 1.5g Fibre - 8.0g	Vit A - 40.59IU Vit B1 (thiamin) - 0.039mg Vit B2 (Riboflavin) - 0.047mg Vit B3 (Niacin) - 0.736mg Vit B6 - 0.068mg Vit C - 32.23mg Folate - 25.83μg Vit E - 1.07mg Vit K - 9.59μg Potassium - 185.73mg Calcium - 30.75mg Phosphorus - 35.67mg Magnesium - 27.06mg	Wash thoroughly in a strainer.

Fruit	Nutritional Value	How to Prepare
Strawberries **152g** **One cup of strawberry halves.** Calories - 49 Protein - 1g Fibre - 3g	Vit A - 18.24IU Vit B1 (thiamin) - 0.036mg Vit B2 (Riboflavin) - 0.033mg Vit B3 (Niacin) - 0.587mg Vit B6 - 0.071mg Vit C - 89.38mg Folate - 36.48µg Vit E - 0.44mg Vit K - 3.34µg Potassium - 232.56mg Calcium - 24.32mg Phosphorus - 36.48mg Magnesium - 19.76mg	Discard the leaf at the top and rinse thoroughly.
Tangerine (Mandarin Orange) **88g** **One medium sized tangerine.** Calories - 46 Protein - 0.7g Fibre - 1.6g	Vit A - 599.28IU Vit B1 (thiamin) - 0.051mg Vit B2 (Riboflavin) - 0.032mg Vit B3 (Niacin) - 0.331mg Vit B6 - 0.069mg Vit C - 23.5mg Folate - 14.08µg Vit E - 0.18mg Vit K - 0.0µg Potassium - 146.08mg Calcium - 32.56mg Phosphorus - 17.6mg Magnesium - 10.56mg	Peel the fruit and divide into segments before placing in the blender.

Fruit	Nutritional Value	How to Prepare
Watermelon **152g** **One cup, diced.** Calories - 46 Protein - 0.9g Fibre - 0.6g	Vit A - 864.88IU Vit B1 (thiamin) - 0.05mg Vit B2 (Riboflavin) - 0.032mg Vit B3 (Niacin) - 0.271mg Vit B6 - 0.068mg Vit C - 12.31mg Folate - 4.56µg Vit E - 0.08mg Vit K - 0.15µg Potassium - 170.24mg Calcium - 10.64mg Phosphorus - 16.72mg Magnesium - 15.2mg	Cut the watermelon into quarters and scoop out the seeds using a small spoon. Peel and discard the rind. Cut the watermelon into diced pieces.

Vegetables	Nutritional Value	How to Prepare
Arugula (Rocket) **20g** **1 cup, chopped.** Calories - 5 Protein - 0.5g Fibre - 0.3g	Vit A - 474.6IU Vit B1 (thiamin) - 0.009mg Vit B2 (Riboflavin) - 0.017mg Vit B3 (Niacin) - 0.061mg Vit B6 - 0.015mg Vit C - 3mg Folate - 19.4µg Vit E - 0.09mg Vit K - 21.72µg Potassium - 73.8mg Calcium - 32mg Phosphorus - 10.4mg Magnesium - 9.4mg	Wash thoroughly and chop.
Asparagus **16g** **1 medium spear.** Calories - 3 Protein - 0.4g Fibre - 0.3g	Vit A - 120.96IU Vit B1 (thiamin) - 0.023mg Vit B2 (Riboflavin) - 0.023mg Vit B3 (Niacin) - 0.156mg Vit B6 - 0.015mg Vit C - 0.9mg Folate - 8.32µg Vit E - 0.18mg Vit K - 6.66µg Potassium - 32.32mg Calcium - 3.84mg Phosphorus - 8.32mg Magnesium - 2.24mg	Wash thoroughly and chop.

Vegetables	Nutritional Value	How to Prepare
Bell Pepper, Green 119g **One medium sized raw sweet green pepper.** Calories - 24 Protein - 1g Fibre - 2g	Vit A - 440.31IU Vit B1 (thiamin) - 0.068mg Vit B2 (Riboflavin) - 0.033mg Vit B3 (Niacin) - 0.571mg Vit B6 - 0.267mg Vit C - 95.68mg Folate - 11.9µg Vit E - 0.44mg Vit K - 8.81µg Potassium - 208.25mg Calcium - 11.9mg Phosphorus - 23.8mg Magnesium - 11.9mg	Remove the stem and wash thoroughly. Chop into small pieces.
Bell Pepper, Red 119g **One medium sized raw sweet red pepper.** Calories - 37 Protein - 1.2g Fibre - 2.5g	Vit A - 3725.89IU Vit B1 (thiamin) - 0.064mg Vit B2 (Riboflavin) - 0.101mg Vit B3 (Niacin) - 1.165mg Vit B6 - 0.346mg Vit C - 151.96mg Folate - 54.74µg Vit E - 1.88mg Vit K - 5.83µg Potassium - 251.09mg Calcium - 8.33mg Phosphorus - 30.94mg Magnesium - 14.28mg	Remove the stem and wash thoroughly. Chop into small pieces.

Vegetables	Nutritional Value	How to Prepare
Beet **82g** **One small sized raw beet.** Calories - 35 Protein - 1.3g Fibre - 2.3g	Vit A - 27.06IU Vit B1 (thiamin) - 0.025mg Vit B2 (Riboflavin) - 0.033mg Vit B3 (Niacin) - 0.274mg Vit B6 - 0.055mg Vit C - 4.02mg Folate - 89.38µg Vit E - 0.03mg Vit K - 0.16µg Potassium - 266.5mg Calcium - 13.12mg Phosphorus - 32.8mg Magnesium - 18.86mg	Peel the fruit to avoid an earthy taste (if you prefer). Cut into small chunks.
Bok Choy (Pak Choy) **70g** **One cup of bok choy, shredded.** Calories - 9 Protein - 1.1g Fibre - 0.7g	Vit A - 3127.6IU Vit B1 (thiamin) - 0.028mg Vit B2 (Riboflavin) - 0.049mg Vit B3 (Niacin) - 0.35mg Vit B6 - 0.136mg Vit C - 31.5mg Folate - 46.2µg Vit E - 0.06mg Vit K - 31.85µg Potassium - 176.4mg Calcium - 73.5mg Phosphorus - 25.9mg Magnesium - 13.3mg	Rinse thoroughly and chop.

Vegetables	Nutritional Value	How to Prepare
Broccoli **31g** **One spear, about 5" long.** Calories - 11 Protein - 0.9g Fibre 0.8g	Vit A - 193.13IU Vit B1 (thiamin) - 0.022mg Vit B2 (Riboflavin) - 0.036mg Vit B3 (Niacin) - 0.198mg Vit B6 - 0.054mg Vit C - 27.65mg Folate - 19.53µg Vit E - 0.24mg Vit K - 31.5µg Potassium - 97.96mg Calcium - 14.57mg Phosphorus - 20.46mg Magnesium - 6.51mg	Wash thoroughly.
Cabbage **89g** **One cup of green cabbage.** Calories - 22 Protein - 1.1g Fibre - 2.2g	Vit A - 87.22IU Vit B1 (thiamin) - 0.054mg Vit B2 (Riboflavin) - 0.036mg Vit B3 (Niacin) - 0.208mg Vit B6 - 0.11mg Vit C - 32.57mg Folate - 38.27µg Vit E - 0.13mg Vit K - 67.64µg Potassium - 151.3mg Calcium - 35.6mg Phosphorus - 23.14mg Magnesium - 10.68mg	Wash the cabbage layers and finely chop into pieces.

Vegetables	Nutritional Value	How to Prepare
Carrot **61g** **One medium sized raw carrot.** Calories - 25 Protein - 0.6g Fibre - 1.7g	Vit A - 10,190.66IU Vit B1 (thiamin) - 0.04mg Vit B2 (Riboflavin) - 0.035mg Vit B3 (Niacin) - 0.6mg Vit B6 - 0.084mg Vit C - 3.6mg Folate - 11.59µg Vit E - 0.4mg Vit K - 8.05µg Potassium - 195.2mg Calcium - 20.13mg Phosphorus - 21.35mg Magnesium - 7.32mg	Wash and scrub thoroughly. Slice before blending.
Celery **40g** **One stalk, medium 7.5 to 8 inches long.** Calories - 6 Protein - 0.3g Fibre - 0.6g	Vit A - 179.6IU Vit B1 (thiamin) - 0.008mg Vit B2 (Riboflavin) - 0.023mg Vit B3 (Niacin) - 0.128mg Vit B6 - 0.03mg Vit C - 1.24mg Folate - 14.4µg Vit E - 0.11mg Vit K - 11.72µg Potassium - 104mg Calcium - 16mg Phosphorus - 9.6mg Magnesium - 4.4mg	Wash thoroughly and slice.

Vegetables	Nutritional Value	How to Prepare
Chard, Swiss 36g **One cup, chopped.** Calories - 7 Protein - 0.6g Fibre - 0.6g	Vit A - 2,201.76IU Vit B1 (thiamin) - 0.014mg Vit B2 (Riboflavin) - 0.032mg Vit B3 (Niacin) - 0.144mg Vit B6 - 0.036mg Vit C - 10.8mg Folate - 5.04µg Vit E - 0.68mg Vit K - 298.8µg Potassium - 136.44mg Calcium - 18.36mg Phosphorus - 16.56mg Magnesium - 29.16mg	Wash thoroughly and chop.
Cherry Tomatoes 149g **One cup of cherry tomatoes.** Calories - 27 Protein - 1.3g Fibre - 1.8g	Vit A - 1241.17IU Vit B1 (thiamin) - 0.055mg Vit B2 (Riboflavin) - 0.028mg Vit B3 (Niacin) - 0.885mg Vit B6 - 0.119mg Vit C - 20.41mg Folate - 22.35µg Vit E - 0.8mg Vit K - 11.77µg Potassium - 353.13mg Calcium - 14.9mg Phosphorus - 35.76mg Magnesium - 16.39mg	Remove stem and any leaves, wash thoroughly and chop.

Vegetables	Nutritional Value	How to Prepare
Collard Greens 36g **One cup of chopped, raw collard greens.** Calories - 12 Protein - 1.1g Fibre - 1.4g	Vit A - 1,806.84IU Vit B1 (thiamin) - 0.019mg Vit B2 (Riboflavin) - 0.047mg Vit B3 (Niacin) - 0.267mg Vit B6 - 0.059mg Vit C - 12.71mg Folate - 46.44µg Vit E - 0.81mg Vit K - 157.36µg Potassium - 76.68mg Calcium - 83.52mg Phosphorus - 9mg Magnesium - 9.72mg	Wash thoroughly and chop.
Cucumber 301g **One medium sized raw cucumber with peel.** Calories - 45 Protein - 2g Fibre - 1.5g	Vit A - 316.05IU Vit B1 (thiamin) - 0.081mg Vit B2 (Riboflavin) - 0.099mg Vit B3 (Niacin) - 0.295mg Vit B6 - 0.12mg Vit C - 8.43mg Folate - 21.07µg Vit E - 0.09mg Vit K - 49.36µg Potassium - 442.47mg Calcium - 48.16mg Phosphorus - 72.24mg Magnesium - 39.13mg	Rinse thoroughly. Cut in half and slice.

Vegetables	Nutritional Value	How to Prepare
Kale **67g** **One cup, chopped.** Calories - 33 Protein - 2.9g Fibre - 2.4g	Vit A - 6693.3IU Vit B1 (thiamin) - 0.074mg Vit B2 (Riboflavin) - 0.087mg Vit B3 (Niacin) - 0.67mg Vit B6 - 0.182mg Vit C - 80.4mg Folate - 94.47µg Vit E - 1.03mg Vit K - 472.2µg Potassium - 328.97mg Calcium - 100.5mg Phosphorus - 61.64mg Magnesium - 31.49mg	Wash thoroughly and chop.
Parsley **60g** **1 cup of chopped parsley.** Calories - 22 Protein - 1.8g Fibre - 2g	Vit A - 5054.4IU Vit B1 (thiamin) - 0.052mg Vit B2 (Riboflavin) - 0.059mg Vit B3 (Niacin) - 0.788mg Vit B6 - 0.054mg Vit C - 79.8mg Folate - 91.2µg Vit E - 0.45mg Vit K - 984µg Potassium - 332.4mg Calcium - 82.8mg Phosphorus - 34.8mg Magnesium - 30mg	Rinse thoroughly and chop.

Vegetables	Nutritional Value	How to Prepare
Romaine Lettuce **47g** **One cup, shredded.** Calories - 8 Protein - 0.6g Fibre - 1g	Vit A - 4,093.7IU Vit B1 (thiamin) - 0.034mg Vit B2 (Riboflavin) - 0.031mg Vit B3 (Niacin) - 0.147mg Vit B6 - 0.035mg Vit C - 1.88mg Folate - 63.92µg Vit E - 0.06mg Vit K - 48.18µg Potassium - 116.09mg Calcium - 15.51mg Phosphorus - 14.1mg Magnesium - 6.58mg	Wash thoroughly and chop.
Spinach **30g** **One cup of raw spinach.** Calories - 7 Protein - 0.9g Fibre - 0.7g	Vit A - 2,813.1IU Vit B1 (thiamin) - 0.023mg Vit B2 (Riboflavin) - 0.057mg Vit B3 (Niacin) - 0.217mg Vit B6 - 0.059mg Vit C - 8.43g Folate - 58.2µg Vit E - 0.61mg Vit K - 144.87µg Potassium - 167.4mg Calcium -29.7mg Phosphorus - 14.7mg Magnesium - 23.7mg	Wash thoroughly.

Vegetables	Nutritional Value	How to Prepare
Tomato **123g** **One medium sized raw tomato.** Calories - 22 Protein - 1.1g Fibre - 1.5g	Vit A - 1024.59IU Vit B1 (thiamin) - 0.046mg Vit B2 (Riboflavin) - 0.023mg Vit B3 (Niacin) - 0.731mg Vit B6 - 0.098mg Vit C - 16.85mg Folate - 18.45µg Vit E - 0.66mg Vit K - 9.72µg Potassium - 291.51mg Calcium - 12.3mg Phosphorus - 29.52mg Magnesium - 13.53mg	Remove stem and any leaves, wash thoroughly and chop.
Watercress **34g** **One cup of chopped watercress.** Calories - 4 Protein - 0.8g Fibre - 0.2g	Vit A - 1084.94IU Vit B1 (thiamin) - 0.031mg Vit B2 (Riboflavin) - 0.041mg Vit B3 (Niacin) - 0.068mg Vit B6 - 0.044mg Vit C - 14.62mg Folate - 3.06µg Vit E - 0.34mg Vit K - 85µg Potassium - 112.2mg Calcium - 40.8mg Phosphorus - 20.4mg Magnesium - 7.14mg	Wash thoroughly and finely chop.

Boosters	Nutritional Value
Acai Powder **15g** **1 tablespoon of freeze-dried acai powder.**	Calories - 28 Protein - 1g Fibre - 2g Fat - 3g Sugar - 0g
Almonds **15g** **1 tablespoon of ground almonds.**	Calories - 81 Protein - 3.3g Fibre - 1.2g Fat - 4.8g Sugar - 0.6g
Almond Milk **250ml** **1 cup.**	Calories - 43 Protein - 1.6g Fibre - 0.9g Fat - 3.8g Sugar - 0.4g
Bee Pollen **2.2g** **1 teaspoon.**	Calories - 16 Protein - 1.2g Fibre - 0.4g Fat - 0.2g Sugar - 1.8g

Boosters	Nutritional Value
Cacao Powder **5g** **1 tablespoon.**	Calories - 11 Protein - 1g Fibre - 1.9g Fat - 0.7g Sugar - 0.1g
Chia Seeds **14g** **1 tablespoon of chia seeds.**	Calories - 60 Protein - 3g Fibre - 6g Fat - 5g Sugar - 0g
Cinnamon **2.6g** **1 teaspoon.**	Calories - 6 Protein - 0.1g Fibre - 1.4g Fat - 0g Sugar - 0.1g
Coconut Oil **Extra Virgin Organic** **3g** **1 teaspoon.**	Calories - 43 Protein - 0g Fibre - 0g Fat - 5g Sugar - 0g

Boosters	Nutritional Value
Coconut Water **250ml** **1 cup.**	Calories - 45 Protein - 0g Fibre - 1g Fat - 0g Sugar - 12.5g
Flax Seed **7g** **1 tablespoon of ground flax seed.**	Calories - 37 Protein - 1.3g Fibre - 1.9g Fat - 3g Sugar - 0.1g
Garlic **3g** **1 garlic clove.**	Calories - 4 Protein - 0.2g Fibre - 0.1g Fat - 0.02g Sugar - 0g
Ginger **11g** **1 inch piece of ginger.**	Calories - 9 Protein - 0.2g Fibre - 0.2g Fat - 0.1g Sugar - 0.2g

Boosters	Nutritional Value
Green Tea **250ml** **1 cup.**	Calories - 2 Protein - 0g Fibre - 0g Fat - 0g Sugar - 0g
Manuka Honey **3g** **1 teaspoon.**	Calories - 5 Protein - 0g Fibre - 0.5g Fat - 0g Sugar - 5g
Mint Leaves **0.1g** **2 leaves.**	Calories - 0 Protein - 0g Fibre - 0g Fat - 0g Sugar - 0g
Pumpkin Seeds **9g** **1 tablespoon of** **pumpkin seeds.**	Calories - 56 Protein - 3g Fibre - 0.6g Fat - 5g Sugar - 0g

Boosters	Nutritional Value
Sesame Seeds **9g** **1 tablespoon of sesame seeds.**	Calories - 52 Protein - 1.6g Fibre - 1.1g Fat - 4.5g Sugar - 0g
Spirulina **2.2g** **1 teaspoon.**	Calories - 7 Protein - 1g Fibre - 0g Fat - 0g Sugar - 0g
Sunflower Sprouts **22g** **¼ cup.**	Calories - 190 Protein - 6g Fibre - 2g Fat - 16g Sugar - 2g
Turmeric, Ground **2.2g** **1 teaspoon.**	Calories - 8 Protein - 0.2g Fibre - 0.5g Fat - 0.02g Sugar - 0.1g

Chapter 6

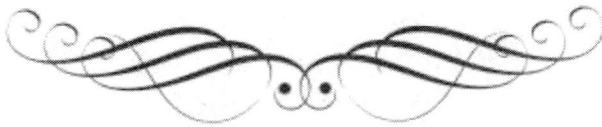

100 Green Smoothie Recipes

Green Fever

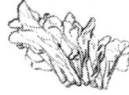

2 cups of kale leaves, stems removed and finely chopped
1 cup of baby spinach
2 pears, peeled and cored
½ inch piece of ginger
1 cup of cooled dandelion tea

Directions
Add the kale and spinach, followed by the pears and ginger. Pour in the dandelion tea to the max line. Add more if necessary. Blend until smooth.

Health Benefits
Reduces the risk of cancer.
Speeds up the elimination of toxins from the blood.
Reduces thickening of the arteries.
Protects against free radical cell damage.

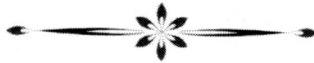

Calories per serving: 281
Yield: 1 Nutribullet cup - 24oz

Berry Green

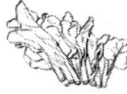

1 cup of arugula
1 cup of parsley, chopped
1 medium celery stalk, chopped
½ cup of blueberries
½ cup of blackberries
½ teaspoon of turmeric
Filtered water

Directions
Add the arugula and parsley, followed by the berries and celery.
Sprinkle in the turmeric powder and pour in the water to the max
line. Blend until smooth.

Health Benefits
Builds and maintains bone strength.
Anti-aging.
Improves digestion.
Wards off bad bacteria from building up in the gut.

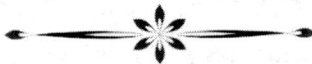

Calories per serving: 110.5
Yield: 1 Nutribullet cup - 24oz

Let Us Be Green

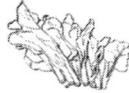

1 cup of romaine lettuce, chopped
1 cup of kale leaves, chopped
1 cup of diced watermelon
1 kiwi fruit, peeled and chopped
1 cup of chilled green tea

Directions

Add the romaine lettuce and kale leaves, followed by the kiwi fruit and watermelon. Pour in the green tea to the max line and add some filtered water if more liquid is required to reach the max line. Blend until smooth.

Health Benefits

Builds a strong immune system.
Ensures healthy growth of cells.
Maintains healthy eyes.
Helps to speed up wound healing.

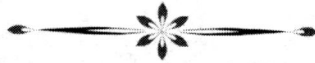

Calories per serving: 131
Yield: 1 Nutribullet cup - 24oz

The Green Goddess

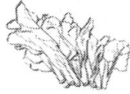

1 cup of Swiss chard
1 cup of spinach
4 broccoli spears
1 apple, cored and chopped
Filtered water

Directions
Add the Swiss chard and spinach, followed by the broccoli and apple.
Pour in the filtered water to the max line and blend until smooth.

Health Benefits
Keeps the skin and tissues hydrated.
Helps with weight loss.
Maintains healthy gums and teeth.
Eliminates toxins from the body.

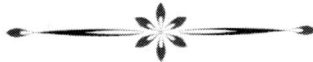

Calories per serving: 153
Yield: 1 Nutribullet cup - 24oz

Green Delight

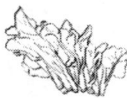

½ cucumber, sliced
½ cup of parsley
2 carrots, sliced
1 ripe banana, chopped
Filtered water

Directions

Add the parsley, followed by the cucumber, carrots, and banana.
Pour in the filtered water to the max line and blend until smooth.

Health Benefits

Promotes radiant, healthy skin.
Prevents against osteoporosis.
Regulates blood sugar levels.
Stimulates a sluggish blood circulation.

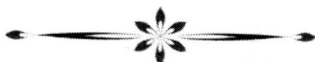

Calories per serving: 188.5
Yield: 1 Nutribullet cup - 24oz

Green Dream

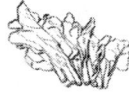

4 broccoli spears
1 cup of watercress
1 pear, cored and chopped
1 kiwi, peeled and sliced
Juice from ½ lemon
Filtered water

Directions

Add the watercress, followed by the broccoli, pear and kiwi. Pour in the lemon juice and filtered water to the max line, and blend until smooth.

Health Benefits

Helps boost metabolism.
Stimulates brain health.
Boosts energy levels.
Protects against cardiovascular disease.

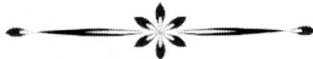

Calories per serving: 196
Yield: 1 Nutribullet cup - 24oz

A Little Taste of Green

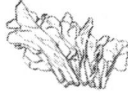

1 cup of spinach
2 carrots, peeled and chopped
2 celery stalks, sliced
½ green bell pepper, cored and chopped
1 cup of chilled green tea

Directions
Add the spinach, followed by the carrots, celery, and green bell pepper. Pour in the green tea to the max line and blend until smooth. Add some filtered water if more liquid is needed to reach the max line.

Health Benefits
Helps to burn fat cells in the body.
Protects the body against disease.
Maintains strong, healthy hair.
Helps to lower blood cholesterol levels.

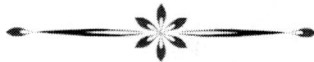

Calories per serving: 83
Yield: 1 Nutribullet cup - 24oz

Green Sunshine

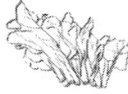

2 cups of dandelion greens
1 banana, sliced
1 cup of pineapple chunks
1 teaspoon of organic coconut oil
Filtered water

Directions

Add the dandelion greens, followed by the banana, pineapple, and coconut oil. Pour in the filtered water to the max line and blend until smooth.

Health Benefits

Helps to delay the signs of aging.
Helps to reduce high blood pressure.
Boosts the immune system.
Maintains healthy joints and muscles.

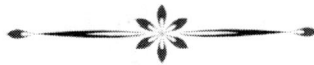

Calories per serving: 280
Yield: 1 Nutribullet cup - 24oz

Green Wonderland

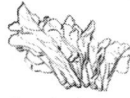

½ cup of parsley, chopped
1 cup of kale, chopped
1 mango, peeled and pitted
½ cup of green seedless grapes
Filtered water

Directions
Add the parsley and kale, followed by the mango and grapes. Pour in the filtered water to the max line and blend until smooth.

Health Benefits
Naturally replenishes lost body fluids.
Stimulates mental clarity and concentration.
Boosts energy levels.
Helps with regular bowel movements.

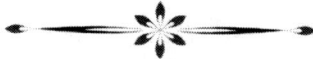

Calories per serving: 195
Yield: 1 Nutribullet cup - 24oz

All You Need is Green

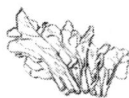

2 cups of watercress
1 orange, peeled and cut up into segments
1 cup of pineapple chunks
1 kiwi, peeled and finely chopped
1 cup of chilled green tea

Directions
Add the watercress followed by the orange, pineapple, and kiwi. Pour in the green tea to the max line and blend until smooth. Add some filtered water if more liquid is neeeded to reach the max line.

Health Benefits
Promotes better sleep.
Soothes inflammation.
Maintains healthy digestion.
Helps with blemishes on the skin.

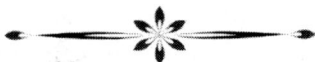

Calories per serving: 196
Yield: 1 Nutribullet cup - 24oz

Glowing Green

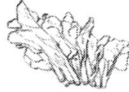

1 cup of romaine lettuce
2 celery stalks, sliced
1 cup of garden peas
1 kiwi, peeled and sliced
Filtered water

Directions
Add the romaine lettuce followed by the celery, peas, and kiwi fruit.
Pour in the filtered water to the max line and blend until smooth.

Health Benefits
Helps to cleanse the blood from impurities.
Protects against urinary tract infections.
Helps to strengthen blood vessels.
Maintains healthy joints and bones.

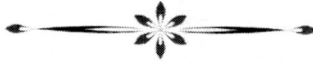

Calories per serving: 180
Yield: 1 Nutribullet cup - 24oz

Green Jingle

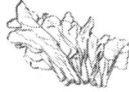

1 cup of spinach
1 carrot, peeled and chopped
1 cup of strawberries, finely chopped
1 cup of cranberries
½ teaspoon of cinnamon
Filtered water

Directions
Add the spinach followed by the carrot, strawberries, and cranberries. Sprinkle in the cinnamon and pour in the filtered water to the max line. Blend until smooth.

Health Benefits
Maintains healthy eye sight.
Combats fluid retention.
Promotes wound healing.
Helps protect against stroke and heart attacks.

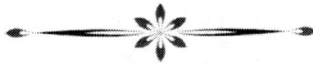

Calories per serving: 130
Yield: 1 Nutribullet cup - 24oz

The Green Mile

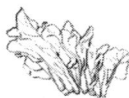

1 cup of dark green cabbage, chopped
1 cup of kale, chopped
½ cup of pineapple chunks
½ cup of raspberries
1 lime, peeled and pitted
1 tablespoon of goji berries
Filtered water

Directions

Add the cabbage and kale, followed by the pineapple, raspberries, lime, and goji berries. Pour in the filtered water to the max line and blend until smooth.

Health Benefits

Promotes healthy cells.
Maintains normal blood pressure.
Maintains a healthy thyroid gland.
Helps to control blood sugar levels.

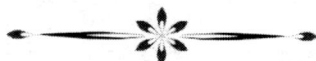

Calories per serving: 177.5
Yield: 1 Nutribullet cup - 24oz

Zingy Green

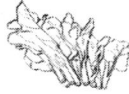

1 red bell pepper, cored and chopped
1 cup of pitted cherries
2 cups of spinach
1 kiwi fruit, peeled and sliced
Filtered water

Directions
Add the spinach, followed by the red bell pepper, cherries, and kiwi fruit. Pour in the filtered water to the max line and blend until smooth.

Health Benefits
Promotes a radiant skin complexion.
Helps to promote a fuller feeling for longer.
Helps to increase the transport of nutrients around the body.
Protects against indigestion.

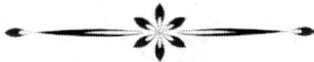

Calories per serving: 190
Yield: 1 Nutribullet cup - 24oz

Ocean Green

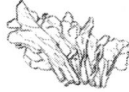

½ cucumber, sliced
1 apple, cored and chopped
1 pear, cored and chopped
1 teaspoon of matcha green tea powder
1 cup of chilled green tea

Directions
Add the cucumber, apple, and pear. Sprinkle in the matcha green tea powder and pour in the green tea to the max line. Add some filtered water if more liquid is needed to reach the max line.

Health Benefits
Speeds up the body's detoxification process.
Helps to improve performance during exercise.
Reduces the risk of getting seasonal colds and flu.
Provides relief from insomnia.

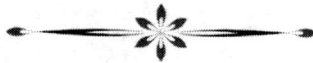

Calories per serving: 224.5
Yield: 1 Nutribullet cup - 24oz

Green Day

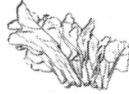

½ avocado, pitted
4 broccoli spears
1 cup of blackcurrants
1 banana, sliced
Filtered water

Directions
Add the avocado, broccoli, banana, and blackcurrants. Pour in the filtered water to the max line and blend until smooth.

Health Benefits
Helps to reduce sugar cravings.
Maintains healthy kidney function.
Protects against cardiovascular disease.
Helps to reduce inflammation.

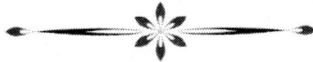

Calories per serving: 381
Yield: 1 Nutribullet cup - 24oz

The Lean Green Fighting Machine

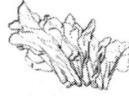

1 cup of kale, chopped
1 cup of romaine lettuce, chopped
1 cup of collard greens
1 apple, cored and chopped
1 kiwi fruit, peeled and sliced
1 tablespoon of chia seeds
Filtered water

Directions

Add the kale, romaine lettuce, and collard greens. Follow with the apple, kiwi fruit, and chia seeds. Pour in the filtered water to the max line and blend until smooth.

Health Benefits

Helps to fight free radical damage.
Helps to maintain a healthy weight.
Prevents against the calcification of arteries.
Relieves feelings of anxiety and depression.

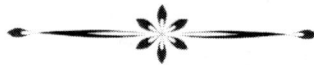

Calories per serving: 250
Yield: 1 Nutribullet cup - 24oz

Everything's Gone Green

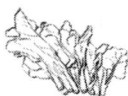

½ cucumber, chopped
2 celery stalks, sliced
1 cup of bok choy, chopped
1 cup of watercress
Juice from 1 lemon
1 cup of chilled nettle tea

Directions
Add the bok choy and watercress, followed by the cucumber and celery. Pour in the lemon juice and nettle tea to the max line, and blend until smooth. Add some filtered water if more liquid is needed to reach the max line.

Health Benefits
Helps to burn fat cells.
Prevents against heart disease.
Stimulates efficient blood circulation.
Improves the appearance of cellulite.

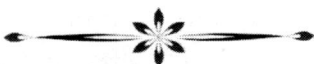

Calories per serving: 57.5
Yield: 1 Nutribullet cup - 24oz

Fried Green Tomatoes

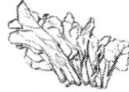

1 green bell pepper, cored and chopped
4 broccoli florets
1 cup of cherry tomatoes
1 teaspoon of spirulina
Filtered water

Directions

Add the green bell pepper, broccoli, and cherry tomatoes. Sprinkle in the spirulina and pour in the filtered water to the max line. Blend until smooth.

Health Benefits

Promotes healthy skin, hair, and nails.
Maintains healthy connective tissue.
Boosts the body's immune system.
Protects cells from free radical damage.

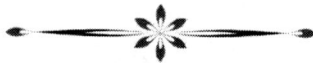

Calories per serving: 102
Yield: 1 Nutribullet cup - 24oz

All About Green

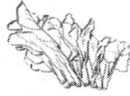

1 cup of spinach
1 pear, cored and chopped
½ cup of green, seedless grapes
¼ cup of sunflower sprouts
1 cup of chilled green tea

Directions
Add the spinach and sprouts, followed by the pear and grapes. Pour in the green tea and blend until smooth. Add some filtered water if more liquid is needed to reach the max line.

Health Benefits
Promotes an energised, refreshed feeling.
Maintains healthy gums.
Helps to ease the symptoms of allergies.
Protects the body's cells and DNA from damage and mutation.

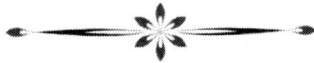

Calories per serving: 353
Yield: 1 Nutribullet cup - 24oz

City Green

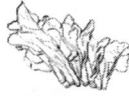

1 cup of kale, chopped
1 cup of spinach
1 beet, peeled and chopped
1 apple, cored and chopped
1 tablespoon of ground flax seed
1 cup of chilled green tea

Directions

Add the kale and spinach, followed by the beet and apple. Sprinkle in the flax seeds and pour in the green tea to the max line. Add some filtered water if more liquid is needed to reach the max line. Blend until smooth.

Health Benefits

Helps to improve brain function.
Reduces the formation of free radicals in the body.
Promotes focus and concentration.
Boosts metabolism.

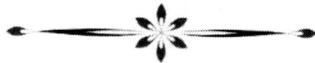

Calories per serving: 209
Yield: 1 Nutribullet cup - 24oz

The Green Rush

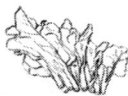

1 cup of dark green cabbage
1 cup of kale
1 cup of dandelion greens
1 banana, sliced
1 cup of pineapple chunks
1 cup of unsweetened or homemade almond milk

Directions
Add the cabbage, kale, and dandelion greens. Follow with the banana and pineapple. Pour in the almond milk to the max line and blend until smooth. Add some filtered water if more liquid is needed to reach the max line.

Health Benefits
Helps to reduce the risk of cancer.
Inhibits the spread of bacteria and viruses.
Helps to reduce bad cholesterol levels in the body.
Promotes healthy weight loss.

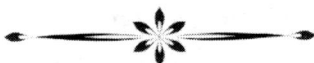

Calories per serving: 310
Yield: 1 Nutribullet cup - 24oz

Green Easy

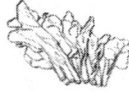

1 apple, cored and chopped
1 pear, cored and chopped
1 kiwi, peeled and sliced
½ cup of green seedless grapes
1 cup of chilled green tea

Directions
Add the apple, pear, kiwi fruit, and grapes. Pour in the green tea to the max line and blend until smooth. Add some filtered water if more liquid is needed to reach the max line.

Health Benefits
Aids in preventing dementia.
Strengthens cardiac muscles.
Maintains healthy bones and joints.
Boosts the immune system.

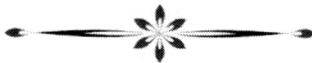

Calories per serving: 293
Yield: 1 Nutribullet cup - 24oz

Green Baby Green

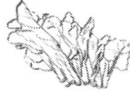

2 cups of spinach
1 carrot, peeled and chopped
½ cucumber, peeled and chopped
½ cup of blueberries
Filtered water

Directions
Add the spinach, followed by the cucumber, carrot, and blueberries.
Pour in the filtered water to the max line and blend until smooth.

Health Benefits
Helps to relieve the symptoms of acne.
Improves memory and concentration.
Prevents against atherosclerosis and strokes.
Promotes a healthy digestive tract.

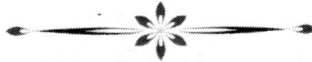

Calories per serving: 103.5
Yield: 1 Nutribullet cup - 24oz

The Big Green

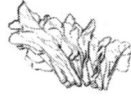

1 cup of watercress
1 pear, cored and chopped
1 peach, pitted
1 tablespoon of goji berries
1 tablespoon of ground flax seed
1 cup of coconut water

Directions
Add the watercress, followed by the pear, peach, and goji berries. Sprinkle in the flaxseeds and pour in the coconut water to the max line. Blend until smooth. If you need to add more liquid, add filtered water so as to avoid extra calories.

Health Benefits
Helps to reduce the symptoms associated with arthritis and rheumatism.
Delays the signs of aging.
Regulates blood sugar levels.
Helps to balance moods.

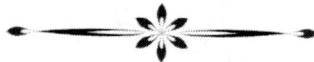

Calories per serving: 276
Yield: 1 Nutribullet cup - 24oz

Paths of Green

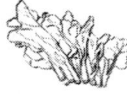

1 cup of kale, chopped
4 broccoli spears
1 cup of strawberries, finely chopped
1 lime, peeled and pitted
1 tablespoon of ground almonds
Filtered water

Directions
Add the kale, followed by the broccoli, strawberries, and lime.
Sprinkle in the ground almonds and pour in the filtered water to the
max line. Blend until smooth.

Health Benefits
Helps to reduce fluid retention and swelling.
Promotes brain health.
Reduces the appearance of fine lines and wrinkles.
Helps to prevent against type 2 diabetes.

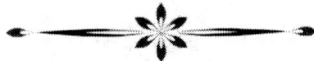

Calories per serving: 227
Yield: 1 Nutribullet cup - 24oz

Darling Buds of Green

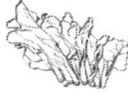

1 apple, cored and chopped
3 asparagus spears, sliced
½ avocado
1 passion fruit
1 teaspoon of matcha green tea powder
Filtered water

Directions
Add the apple, asparagus, avocado, and passion fruit. Sprinkle in the matcha green tea powder and pour in the filtered water to the max line. Blend until smooth.

Health Benefits
Helps to relieve dandruff, promoting a healthy scalp.
Protects against colds and flu.
Reduces uric acid build up in joints.
Helps to lower high blood pressure.

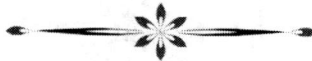

Calories per serving: 285
Yield: 1 Nutribullet cup - 24oz

Top Green

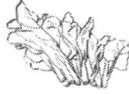

4 broccoli spears
1 papaya, pitted and chopped
1 celery stalk, sliced
1 teaspoon of bee pollen
1 cup of chilled chamomile tea

Directions
Add the broccoli, papaya, and celery. Sprinkle in the bee pollen and pour in the chamomile tea to the max line. Add some filtered water if more liquid is needed to reach the max line. Blend until smooth.

Health Benefits
Helps to rejuvenate skin cells.
Provides relief against constipation.
Promotes healthy gums and teeth.
Acts as a tonic for the liver and gall bladder.

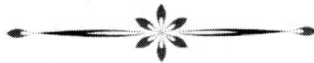

Calories per serving: 135
Yield: 1 Nutribullet cup - 24oz

Pulp Green

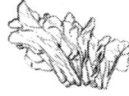

2 cups of Swiss chard, chopped
1 cup of strawberries, finely chopped
1 banana, sliced
½ cup of cranberries
Filtered water

Directions
Add the Swiss chard, followed by the strawberries, banana, and cranberries. Pour in the filtered water to the max line and blend until smooth.

Health Benefits
Helps to improve the appearance of varicose veins.
Reduces acidity in the body.
Anti-inflammatory.
Speeds up the healing of wounds and sores.

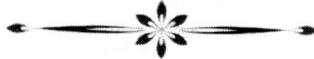

Calories per serving: 191
Yield: 1 Nutribullet cup - 24oz

The Green Tiger

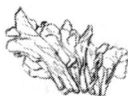

1 cup of watercress
½ cup of fresh parsley, chopped
2 tomatoes, chopped
1 peach, pitted
Juice from ½ lemon
1 cup of chilled green tea

Directions
Add the watercress and parsley. Follow with the tomatoes and peach. Pour in the lemon juice and green tea to the max line. Blend until smooth. Add some filtered water if more liquid is needed to reach the max line.

Health Benefits
Promotes healthy, glowing skin.
Reduces red, inflamed, puffy skin.
Acts as a tonic for the kidneys.
Helps to increase red blood cell count.

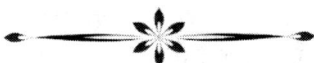

Calories per serving: 123
Yield: 1 Nutribullet cup - 24oz

Green Glory

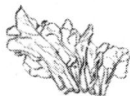

1 cup of kale leaves, finely chopped
1 cup of strawberries, finely chopped
½ cup of red, seedless grapes
1 carrot, peeled and chopped
1 cup of chilled green tea

Directions
Add the kale, followed by the strawberries, grapes, and carrot. Pour in the green tea to the max line and blend until smooth. Add some filtered water if more liquid is needed to reach the max line.

Health Benefits
Reduces free radical damage to cells.
Stimulates hair growth.
Prevents kidney infections.
Accelerates wound healing.

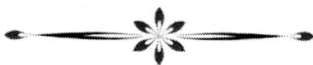

Calories per serving: 161
Yield: 1 Nutribullet cup - 24oz

Green River

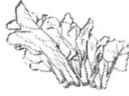

1 cup of spinach
1 cup of bok choy, finely chopped
1 orange, peeled and cut into segments
½ cup of dark, pitted frozen cherries
1 tablespoon of chia seeds
Filtered water

Directions
Add the spinach and bok choy, followed by the orange, cherries, and chia seeds. Pour in the filtered water to the max line and blend until smooth.

Health Benefits
Reduces the risk of allergic reactions.
Maintains healthy blood pressure levels.
Reduces the appearance of fine line and wrinkles.
Improves digestive health.

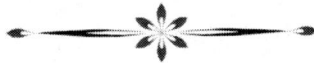

Calories per serving: 186.5
Yield: 1 Nutribullet cup - 24oz

The Green Wizard

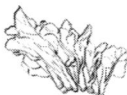

2 cups of Swiss chard, finely chopped
1 green apple, cored and chopped
½ cup of green, seedless grapes
1 kiwi, peeled and finely chopped
Filtered water

Directions
Add the Swiss chard, followed by the apple, grapes, and kiwi fruit.
Pour in the filtered water to the max line and blend until smooth.

Health Benefits
Stimulates hair growth.
Helps to relieve stress and pressure on blood vessels.
Alleviates dry skin conditions such as psoriasis and cracked skin.
Helps to defend the body against foreign pathogens and agents.

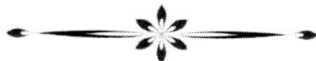

Calories per serving: 203
Yield: 1 Nutribullet cup - 24oz

Green Heights

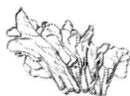

½ cucumber, finely chopped
1 avocado, chopped and pitted
1 apple, cored
1 cup of chilled green tea

Directions

Add the cucumber, avocado, and apple. Pour in the green tea to the max line and blend until smooth. Add some filtered water if more liquid is needed to reach the max line.

Health Benefits

Helps to prevent against rheumatoid arthritis.
Helps regulate menstruation.
Purifies blood.
Improves skin elasticity and firmness.

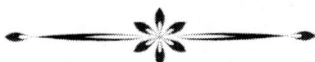

Calories per serving: 441.5
Yield: 1 Nutribullet cup - 24oz

Green Paradise

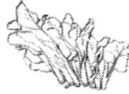

1 green bell pepper, cored and chopped
1 pear, cored
1 beet, peeled and chopped
½ teaspoon of cinnamon
1 tablespoon of ground flax seed
1 cup of coconut water

Directions
Add the green pepper, pear, and beet. Sprinkle in the cinnamon and ground flax seed, and pour in the coconut water. Blend until smooth. Add filtered water if more liquid is needed to reach the max line.

Health Benefits
Regulates blood sugar levels.
Improves red blood cell count.
Reduces bad cholesterol levels.
Helps with healthy weight loss.

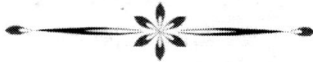

Calories per serving: 246
Yield: 1 Nutribullet cup - 24oz

Green Rebel

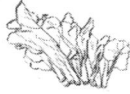

1 cup of spinach
5 broccoli spears
1 celery stalk, chopped
2 lemon wedges
Filtered water

Directions
Add the spinach, broccoli, celery, and lemon. Pour in the filtered water to the max line and blend until smooth.

Health Benefits
Neutralises acidity in the blood.
Replaces lost electrolytes in the body.
Decreases the chances of constipation.
Eliminates fluid retention.

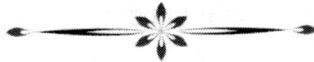

Calories per serving: 72
Yield: 1 Nutribullet cup - 24oz

The Green Story

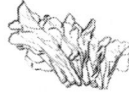

1 cup of spinach
1 carrot, peeled and chopped
1 banana, sliced
1 tablespoon of sesame seeds
1 teaspoon of coconut oil
1 cup of chilled green tea

Directions
Add the spinach, carrot, and banana. Sprinkle in the sesame seeds and add the coconut oil. Pour in the green tea and blend until smooth. Add some filtered water if more liquid is needed to reach the max line.

Health Benefits
Reduces the risk of cancer.
Helps to lower high blood pressure.
Reduces inflamed joints.
Boosts energy levels.

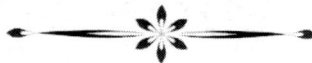

Calories per serving: 234
Yield: 1 Nutribullet cup - 24oz

A Touch of Green

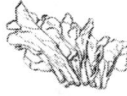

2 cups of romaine lettuce, finely chopped
1 cup of kale, finely chopped
1 banana, sliced
1 kiwi fruit, peeled and chopped
1 tablespoon of ground almonds
Filtered water

Directions
Add the romaine lettuce, kale, banana, and kiwi fruit. Sprinkle in the ground almonds and pour in the filtered water to the max line. Blend until smooth.

Health Benefits
Reduces the appearance of age spots.
Helps to combat anaemia.
Improves the appearance of wrinkles and skin tone.
Maintains eye health.

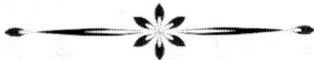

Calories per serving: 277
Yield: 1 Nutribullet cup - 24oz

Green Mission

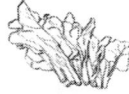

1 cup of parsley, finely chopped
2 ripe pears, cored and chopped
2 lemon wedges
1 teaspoon of spirulina
1 cup of chilled nettle tea

Directions
Add the parsley, pears, and lemon wedges. Sprinkle in the spirulina and pour in the nettle tea. Add some filtered water if more liquid is needed to reach the max line. Blend until smooth.

Health Benefits
Reduces skin inflammation.
Provides relief from PMS.
Protects against bacterial and viral infections.
Enhances brain health.

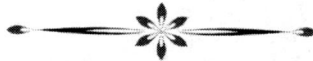

Calories per serving: 239
Yield: 1 Nutribullet cup - 24oz

Something Green

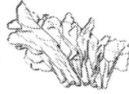

1 cup of watercress
1 orange, peeled and cut into segments
1 cup of blueberries
1 carrot, peeled and chopped
Filtered water

Directions
Add the watercress, orange, blueberries, and carrot. Pour in the filtered water to the max line and blend until smooth.

Health Benefits
Helps to heal dry skin conditions such as eczema and psoriasis.
Helps to reduce stress levels.
Provides relief from insomnia.
Hydrates the skin.

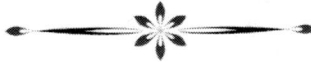

Calories per serving: 175
Yield: 1 Nutribullet cup - 24oz

The Green Engagement

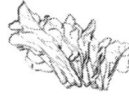

1 stalk of celery, finely chopped
1 cup of dandelion greens
1 banana, sliced
½ cup of red seedless grapes
Filtered water

Directions
Add the dandelion greens, followed by the celery, banana, and grapes.
Pour in the filtered water to the max line and blend until smooth.

Health Benefits
Provides relief from heartburn.
Acts as a tonic for healthy digestion.
Helps to eliminate toxins from the body.
Promotes healthy gums and teeth.

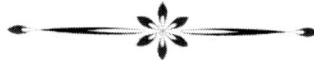

Calories per serving: 188
Yield: 1 Nutribullet cup - 24oz

The Green Adventure

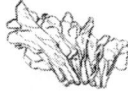

1 cup of spinach
2 kiwi fruit, peeled and chopped
½ cucumber, finely chopped
1 peach, pitted and chopped
Filtered water

Directions
Add the spinach, followed by the kiwi fruit, cucumber, and peach.
Pour in the filtered water to the max line and blend until smooth.

Health Benefits
Keeps tissues and skin hydrated.
Promotes radiant, healthy skin.
Reduces puffy eyes.
Helps to prevent urinary tract infections.

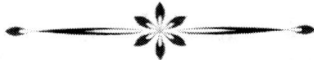

Calories per serving: 172.5
Yield: 1 Nutribullet cup - 24oz

Green Emerald

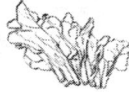

4 broccoli spears
1 cup of diced watermelon
2 asparagus spears, chopped
½ inch piece of ginger
Filtered water

Directions
Add the broccoli, watermelon, asparagus, and ginger. Pour in the filtered water to the max line and blend until smooth.

Health Benefits
Lowers the risk of atherosclerosis.
Reduces the appearance of varicose veins.
Strengthens blood vessels.
Stimulates healthy digestion.

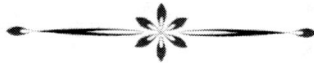

Calories per serving: 105
Yield: 1 Nutribullet cup - 24oz

Green Feast

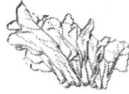

2 cups of dandelion greens, finely chopped
½ cucumber, sliced
1 cup of strawberries, finely chopped
1 lemon wedge
1 cup of chilled green tea

Directions

Add the dandelion greens, followed by the cucumber, strawberries, and lemon. Pour in the green tea and blend until smooth. Add some filtered water if more liquid is needed to reach the max line.

Health Benefits

Maintains healthy tissue and cartilage.
Regulates bowel movement.
Helps burn stored fat.
Protects elastin fibres from damage, reducing sagging skin.

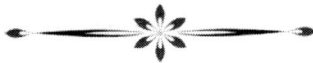

Calories per serving: 125.5
Yield: 1 Nutribullet cup - 24oz

Green Beauty

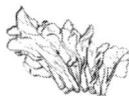

1 cup of spinach
1 cup of green seedless grapes
1 mango, peeled and pitted
1 tablespoon of cacao powder
Filtered water

Directions
Add the spinach, followed by the grapes and mango. Sprinkle in the cacao powder and pour in the filtered water to the max line. Blend until smooth.

Health Benefits
Boosts short term memory.
Reduces the risk of heart disease.
Anti-inflammatory.
Promotes strong hair and nails.

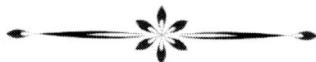

Calories per serving: 221
Yield: 1 Nutribullet cup - 24oz

Green Velvet

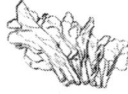

2 cups of kale leaves, finely chopped
1 pear, cored and chopped
1 beet, peeled and chopped
1 kiwi fruit, peeled and chopped
Filtered water

Directions

Add the kale leaves, followed by the pear, beet, and kiwi fruit. Pour in the filtered water to the max line and blend until smooth.

Health Benefits

Helps to increase muscle strength.
Reduces mood swings.
Reduces the risk of arthritis.
Maintains a healthy digestive tract.

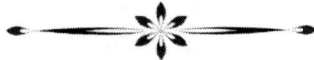

Calories per serving: 245
Yield: 1 Nutribullet cup - 24oz

Green Celebration

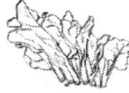

1 cup of romaine lettuce, finely chopped
1 apple, cored and chopped
1 cup of raspberries
½ cup of cherries, pitted
1 cup of coconut water

Directions
Add the romaine lettuce, followed by the apple, raspberries, and cherries. Pour in the coconut water and blend until smooth. Add some filtered water if more liquid is needed to reach the max line.

Health Benefits
Reduces the symptoms of irritable bowel syndrome.
Lowers bad cholesterol levels.
Strengthens the immune system.
Maintains healthy brain function.

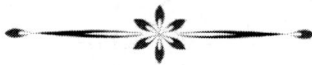

Calories per serving: 261.5
Yield: 1 Nutribullet cup - 24oz

The Green Dozen

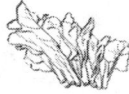

1 cup of kale, finely chopped
1 cup of spinach
1 banana, chopped
1 peach, pitted and chopped
1 cup of chilled green tea

Directions
Add the kale and spinach, followed by the banana and peach. Pour in the green tea and blend until smooth. Add some filtered water if more liquid is needed to reach the max line.

Health Benefits
Helps to regulate blood pressure.
Maintains healthy bones and joints.
Helps to reduce cellulite.
Increases the absorption of nutrients in the blood.

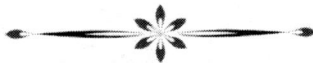

Calories per serving: 206
Yield: 1 Nutribullet cup - 24oz

Fifty Shades of Green

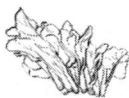

1 cup of romaine lettuce
3 asparagus spears, chopped
½ cucumber, sliced
1 cup of pineapple chunks
½ teaspoon of ground turmeric
Filtered water

Directions

Add the romaine lettuce, followed by the asparagus, cucumber, and pineapple. Sprinkle in the ground turmeric and pour in the filtered water to the max line. Blend until smooth.

Health Benefits

Protects cells from oxidative damage.
Helps to protect against osteoporosis.
Reduces the symptoms of PMS and menopause.
Increases skin regeneration.

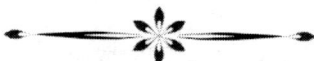

Calories per serving: 125.5
Yield: 1 Nutribullet cup - 24oz

Bring on the Green

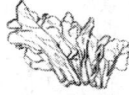

4 broccoli florets
1 celery stalk, chopped
1 tomato, chopped into small chunks
1 red bell pepper, cored and chopped into chunks
Filtered water

Directions
Add the broccoli, celery, tomato, and red bell pepper. Pour in the
filtered water to the max line and blend until smooth.

Health Benefits
Helps to fight against free radical damage.
Promotes regular urination and bowel movement.
Maintains the body's electrolyte balance.
Reduces the risk of coronary heart disease.

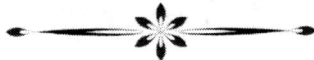

Calories per serving: 109
Yield: 1 Nutribullet cup - 24oz

The Green Takeaway

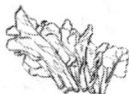

1 cup of spinach
1 cup of watercress
1 cup of Swiss chard
1 celery stalk
1 cup of blueberries
1 tablespoon of ground flax seeds
Filtered water

Directions

Add the spinach, watercress, and Swiss chard, followed by the celery and blueberries. Sprinkle in the ground flax seeds and pour in the filtered water to the max line. Blend until smooth.

Health Benefits

Stimulates a healthy digestive tract.
Reduces the risk of cancer.
Promotes a healthy skin complexion.
Accelerates the healing of cuts and wounds.

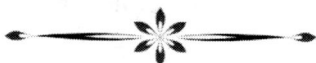

Calories per serving: 145
Yield: 1 Nutribullet cup - 24oz

Energise Green

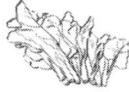

½ cup of parsley, finely chopped
1 beet, peeled and finely chopped
2 apples, cored and chopped
1 kiwi, peeled and chopped
1 cup of chilled green tea

Directions
Add the parsley, followed by the beet, apples, and kiwi. Pour in the green tea and blend until smooth. Add some filtered water if more liquid is needed to reach the max line.

Health Benefits
Reduces respiratory problems such as asthma and bronchitis.
Acts as a tonic for the liver and gall bladder.
Soothes the nervous system.
Promotes a peaceful night's sleep.

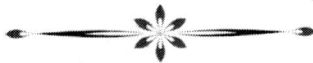

Calories per serving: 280
Yield: 1 Nutribullet cup - 24oz

Healthy Green Water

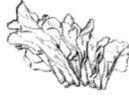

2 cups of romaine lettuce
1 cup of diced watermelon
½ cup of cranberries
2 mint leaves, finely chopped
1 tablespoon of sesame seeds
Filtered water

Directions
Add the romaine lettuce, followed by the watermelon, cranberries, and mint. Sprinkle in the ssesame seeds and pour in the filtered water to the max line. Blend until smooth.

Health Benefits
Reduces feelings of anxiety and tension in the body.
Helps to reduce inflammation around joints.
Improves focus and mental alertness.
Increases energy levels.

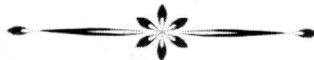

Calories per serving: 137
Yield: 1 Nutribullet cup - 24oz

"G" is for Green

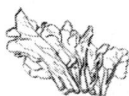

4 broccoli spears
1 cup of spinach
1 cup of blackberries
1 mango, pitted and chopped
1 cup of chilled chamomile tea

Directions
Add the spinach, followed by the broccoli, blackberries, and mango.
Pour in the chamomile tea and blend until smooth. Add some
filtered water if more liquid is needed to reach the max line.

Health Benefits
Reduces the appearance of fine lines and wrinkles.
Helps to repair damaged connective tissue.
Helps to eliminate toxins and wastes from the body.
Alkalises the body and blood.

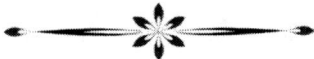

Calories per serving: 214
Yield: 1 Nutribullet cup - 24oz

Spicy Green

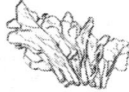

2 kiwi fruit, peeled and chopped
1 apple, cored and chopped
1 pear, cored and chopped
1 celery stalk, chopped
1 cup of chilled green tea

Directions
Add the kiwi fruit, apple, pear, and celery. Pour in the green tea, adding some filtered water if more liquid is needed to reach the max line. Blend until smooth.

Health Benefits
Keeps the skin cells hydrated.
Reduces the risk of heart disease.
Anti-aging.
Reduces reaction to allergies.

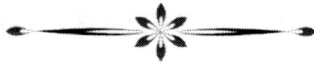

Calories per serving: 289
Yield: 1 Nutribullet cup - 24oz

Elegant Green

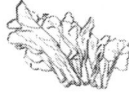

1 cup of romaine lettuce, finely chopped
1 cup of spinach leaves
½ cup of pineapple chunks
1 apple, cored and chopped
Filtered water

Directions
Add the romaine lettuce and spinach, followed by the pineapple and apple. Pour in the filtered water to the max line and blend until smooth.

Health Benefits
Helps to protect against colds and flu.
Reduces bad cholesterol levels.
Helps to melt fat cells.
Strengthens the lining of blood vessels.

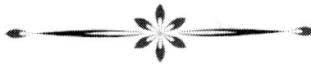

Calories per serving: 151
Yield: 1 Nutribullet cup - 24oz

Mushy Green

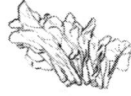

1 cup of arugula
4 broccoli spears
1 cup of pitted cherries
1 cup of blackcurrants
1 cup of coconut water

Directions

Add the arugula, followed by the broccoli, cherries, and blackcurrants.
Pour in the coconut water and blend until smooth. Add some filtered
water if more liquid is needed to reach the max line.

Health Benefits

Reduces fatigue and mental exhaustion.
Protects the skin from free radical damage.
Maintains healthy kidney function.
Promotes healthy production of red blood cells.

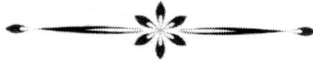

Calories per serving: 262
Yield: 1 Nutribullet cup - 24oz

Mystery Green

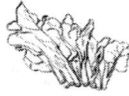

4 broccoli spears
1 cup of spinach
½ avocado
2 plums, pitted and chopped
Filtered water

Directions
Add the spinach, followed by the broccoli, avocado, and plums. Pour in the filtered water to the max line and blend until smooth.

Health Benefits
Controls sebum production on oily skin.
Regulates blood sugar levels.
Aids with weight loss.
Helps to detoxify the body.

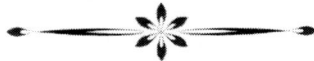

Calories per serving: 272
Yield: 1 Nutribullet cup - 24oz

Easy Green

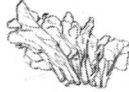

1 cup of collard greens, finely chopped
2 celery stalks, chopped
1 carrot, peeled and sliced
1 green bell pepper, cored and chopped
1 cup of chilled green tea

Directions
Add the collard greens, followed by the celery, carrot, and green bell pepper. Pour in the green tea to the max line and blend until smooth. Add some filtered water if more liquid is needed to reach the max line.

Health Benefits
Stimulates blood circulation.
Improves cognitive function.
Keeps the skin supple and strong.
Reduces the build up of plaque around arteries.

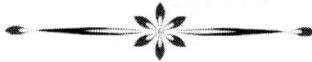

Calories per serving: 75
Yield: 1 Nutribullet cup - 24oz

The Green Blues

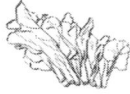

1 cup of dandelion greens
1 cup of cherry tomatoes
1 apple, cored and chopped
1 tablespoon of ground almonds
1 cup of coconut water

Directions

Add the dandelion greens, followed by the cherry tomatoes and apple.
Sprinkle in the ground almonds and pour in the coconut water.
Blend until smooth. Add some filtered water if more liquid is needed
to reach the max line.

Health Benefits

Promotes healthy calcium absorption.
Maintains lean body mass.
Healthy production of antibodies, hormones, and enzymes.
Stimulates collagen formation in the skin.

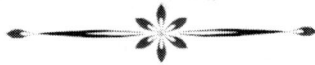

Calories per serving: 273
Yield: 1 Nutribullet cup - 24oz

Whole Lotta' Green

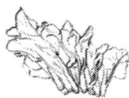

1 cup of spinach
½ cup of parsley, chopped
2 kiwi's, peeled and chopped
1 orange, peeled, pitted and cut into segments
Filtered water

Directions
Add the spinach and parsley, followed by the kiwi fruit and orange.
Pour in the filtered water to the max line and blend until smooth.

Health Benefits
Provides relief from sinusitis.
Reduces inflammation in joints and muscles.
Helps to reduce the accumulation of fat in the liver.
Helps to maintain normal heart function.

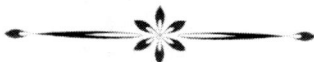

Calories per serving: 164
Yield: 1 Nutribullet cup - 24oz

Green Dreamin'

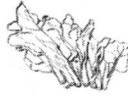

2 cups of spinach
1 cup of strawberries, finely chopped
1 banana, sliced
1 tablespoon of ground flax seed
1 cup of almond milk

Directions

Add the spinach, followed by the strawberries and banana. Sprinkle in the ground flax seed and pour in the almond milk. Blend until smooth. Add some filtered water if more liquid is needed to reach the max line.

Health Benefits

Stimulates haemoglobin and red cell production.
Promotes health female and male reproduction.
Acts as a diuretic.
Maintains normal immune function.

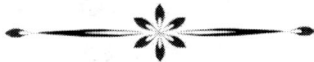

Calories per serving: 241
Yield: 1 Nutribullet cup - 24oz

Green Haze

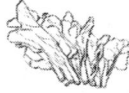

1 cup of watercress
1 celery stalk, chopped
½ cucumber, sliced
½ cup of pitted cherries
Filtered water

Directions
Add the watercress, followed by the celery, cucumber, and cherries.
Pour in the filtered water to the max line and blend until smooth.

Health Benefits
Promotes collagen production and tissue repair.
Maintains healthy blood pressure levels.
Promotes respiratory tract health.
Reduces the risk of cancer.

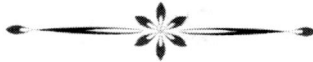

Calories per serving: 81
Yield: 1 Nutribullet cup - 24oz

Go the Green Way

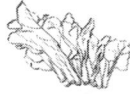

1 cup of dark green cabbage, finely chopped
4 asparagus spears, finely sliced
½ red bell pepper, cored and chopped
½ cup of cranberries
Filtered water

Directions
Add the cabbage, followed by the asparagus, cranberries, and red bell pepper. Pour in the filtered water to the max line and blend until smooth.

Health Benefits
Prevents against bacterial infections.
Reduces muscle cramps.
Promotes healthy red blood cell production.
Promotes healthy adrenal gland function.

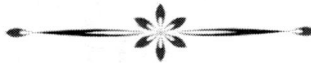

Calories per serving: 75.5
Yield: 1 Nutribullet cup - 24oz

Chitty Green Bang Bang

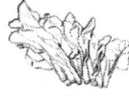

1 cup of spinach
1 cup of parsley, chopped
½ cup of green seedless grapes
½ cup of watermelon, diced
1 tablespoon of goji berries
1 cup of chilled green tea

Add the spinach and parsley, followed by the grapes, watermelon, and goji berries. Pour in the green tea and blend until smooth. Add some filtered water if more liquid is needed to reach the max line.

Health Benefits
Maintains healthy reproduction organs.
Lowers high blood pressure.
Reduces bad cholesterol levels.
Anti-inflammatory.

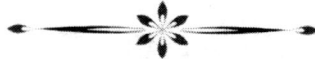

Calories per serving: 135
Yield: 1 Nutribullet cup - 24oz

Green Tutti Fruitti

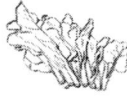

2 cup of kale, finely chopped
1 mango, peeled and pitted
1 banana, sliced
½ teaspoon of cinnamon
Filtered water

Directions
Add the kale, followed by the mango and banana. Sprinkle in the cinnamon and pour in the filtered water to the max line. Blend until smooth.

Health Benefits
Helps to improve blood flow.
Reduces inflammation in bones and joints.
Promotes healthy blood clotting.
Reduces symptoms of allergies.

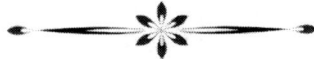

Calories per serving: 273
Yield: 1 Nutribullet cup - 24oz

Green Satisfaction

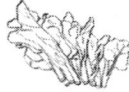

1 cup of spinach
2 broccoli spears
1 pear, cored and chopped
1 apple, cored and chopped
1 cup of coconut water

Directions
Add the spinach, followed by the broccoli, pear, and apple. Pour in the coconut water and blend until smooth. Add some filtered water if more liquid is needed to reach the max line.

Health Benefits
Enhances energy production within cells.
Helps to regulate normal metabolism.
Maintains the health and structure of the skin.
Reduces the symptoms of acne and blemished skin.

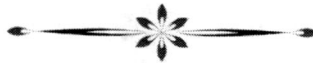

Calories per serving: 271
Yield: 1 Nutribullet cup - 24oz

The Green Hound Dog

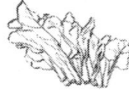

1 cup of bok choy, finely chopped
2 peaches, pitted and chopped
1 cup of blueberries
1 tablespoon of pumpkin seeds
Filtered water

Directions
Add the bok choy, followed by the peaches and blueberries. Sprinkle
in the pumpkin seeds and pour in the filtered water to the max line.
Blend until smooth.

Health Benefits
Maintains healthy thyroid hormone manufacture.
Alleviates dry skin conditions such as psoriasis.
Stimulates healthy nerve cell function.
Protects against damage to cell membranes.

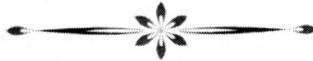

Calories per serving: 267
Yield: 1 Nutribullet cup - 24oz

Heard it Through the Greenvine

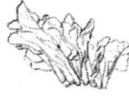

1 cup of spinach
1 green bell pepper, cored and chopped
1 lime, peeled and chopped
1 banana, chopped
Filtered water

Directions
Add the spinach, followed by the green bell pepper, lime, and banana.
Pour in the filtered water to the max line and blend until smooth.

Health Benefits
Maintains healthy protein levels in the body.
Prevents against osteoporosis.
Healthy vision.
Promotes healthy mucus membranes.

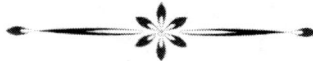

Calories per serving: 156
Yield: 1 Nutribullet cup - 24oz

Rolling Green

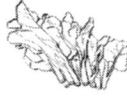

1 cup of dandelion greens, finely chopped
2 celery stalks, sliced
1 cup of strawberries, finely chopped
1 cup of watermelon, diced
1 cup of chilled green tea

Directions

Add the dandelion greens, followed by the celery stalks, strawberries, and watermelon. Pour in the green tea and blend until smooth. Add some filtered water if more liquid is needed to reach the max line.

Health Benefits

Helps to reduce stress levels.
Promotes healthy hair and nails.
Stimulates skin regeneration.
Delays the signs of aging.

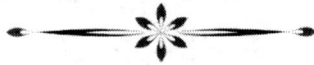

Calories per serving: 134
Yield: 1 Nutribullet cup - 24oz

Stairway to Green

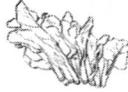

1 cup of spinach
1 papaya, pitted and chopped
½ cup of pineapple chunks
1 passion fruit
Filtered water

Directions
Add the spinach, followed by the papaya, pineapple, and passion fruit.
Pour in the filtered water to the max line and blend until smooth.

Health Benefits
Helps to prevents respiratory tract disorders.
Reduces the risk of cardiovascular disease.
Combats oxidative damage to cells.
Speeds up the healing of bacterial infections.

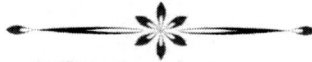

Calories per serving: 132
Yield: 1 Nutribullet cup - 24oz

The Green Prayer

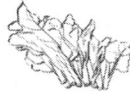

1 cup of dark green cabbage, finely chopped
1 kiwi, peeled and chopped
1 pear, peeled and cored
1 tablespoon of ground flax seed
1 teaspoon of manuka honey
Filtered water

Directions
Add the cabbage, followed by the kiwi fruit and pear. Sprinkle in the ground flax seed and manuka honey. Pour in the filtered water to the max line and blend until smooth.

Health Benefits
Reduces cellular DNA damage.
Reduces the risk of heart disease and strokes.
Protects against common colds.
Promotes the effects of exercise.

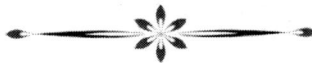

Calories per serving: 208
Yield: 1 Nutribullet cup - 24oz

Too Green For School

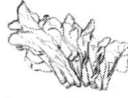

1 cup of parsley, chopped
1 cup of spinach
1 celery stalk
½ cucumber, sliced
1 lime, peeled and chopped
1 tablespoon of organic coconut oil
1 cup of coconut water

Directions

Add the parsley and spinach, followed by the celery, cucumber, and lime. Pour in the coconut oil and coconut water. Blend until smooth. Add some filtered water if more liquid is needed to reach the max line.

Health Benefits

Maintains healthy connective tissue.
Supports the structure of tissues and organs.
Promotes collagen production.
Promotes healthy iron absorption in the body.

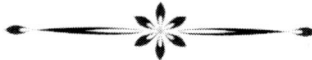

Calories per serving: 165.5
Yield: 1 Nutribullet cup - 24oz

The Green Rose

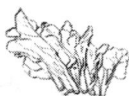

2 cups of spinach
1 kiwi, peeled and cut into chunks
2 mint leaves, finely chopped
1 cup of pineapple chunks
Filtered water

Directions

Add the spinach and mint leaves, followed by the kiwi fruit and pineapple. Pour in the filtered water to the max line and blend until smooth.

Health Benefits

Increases energy levels.
Maintains healthy gums and teeth.
Speeds up wound healing.
Promotes healthy eyes and vision.

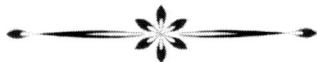

Calories per serving: 138
Yield: 1 Nutribullet cup - 24oz

Green Shack

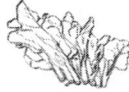

2 cups of kale, finely chopped
1 cup of arugula
1 pear, cored and chopped
1 papaya, cored and chopped
½ inch piece of ginger
Filtered water

Directions
Add the kale and arugula, followed by the pear, papaya, and ginger.
Pour in the filtered water to the max line and blend until smooth.

Health Benefits
Promotes the healthy production of neurotransmitters.
Boosts the immune system.
Facilitates the growth of healthy connective tissue.
Maintains proper brain function.

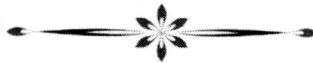

Calories per serving: 244.5
Yield: 1 Nutribullet cup - 24oz

The Green Look

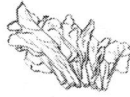

1 cup of spinach
3 broccoli spears
1 carrot, peeled and chopped
1 apple, cored and chopped
1 tablespoon of chia seeds
1 cup of chilled green tea

Directions

Add the spinach, followed by the broccoli, carrot, apple, and chia seeds. Pour in the green tea and blend until smooth. Add some filtered water if more liquid is needed to reach the max line.

Health Benefits

Aids in lowering high blood pressure.
Reduces the risk of cancer.
Helps to reduce the symptoms of asthma.
Helps to control diabetes.

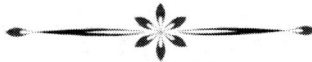

Calories per serving: 222
Yield: 1 Nutribullet cup - 24oz

Green Breath

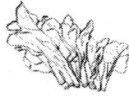

2 cups of kale, finely chopped
1 cup of pitted cherries
1 peach, pitted
½ cup of melon cubes
1 teaspoon of spirulina
Filtered water

Directions

Add the kale, followed by the cherries, peach, and melon. Sprinkle in the spirulina and pour in the filtered water to the max line. Blend until smooth.

Health Benefits

Healthy skin and eyes.
Acts as a tonic for the lungs.
Helps to prevent against arthritis.
Helps to decrease stress levels in the body.

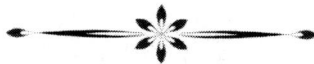

Calories per serving: 256
Yield: 1 Nutribullet cup - 24oz

Sweet Green Dreams

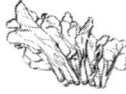

1 cup of green cabbage, finely chopped
1 banana, sliced
1 apple, cored and chopped
1 tablespoon of cacao powder
1 cup of coconut water

Directions

Add the cabbage, followed by the banana and apple. Sprinkle in the cacao powder and pour in the coconut water. Blend until smooth. Pour in some filtered water if more liquid is needed to reach the max line.

Health Benefits

Aids in improving insulin metabolism.
Reduces the risk of gastrointestinal disorders.
Protects the skin against harmful toxins.
Helps to reduce inflammation and protect against arthritis.

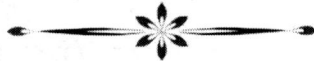

Calories per serving: 278
Yield: 1 Nutribullet cup - 24oz

Green Superhero

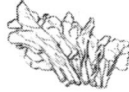

1 cup of spinach
¼ cup of sunflower sprouts
1 cup of green seedless grapes
1 kiwi, peeled and chopped
1 carrot, peeled and sliced
Filtered water

Directions
Add the spinach and sprouts, followed by the grapes, kiwi, and carrot.
Pour in the filtered water to the max line and blend until smooth.

Health Benefits
Relieves the symptoms of stress and anxiety.
Helps to speed up the metabolic rate.
Protects against fungal infections such as athlete's foot.
Stimulates cell regeneration.

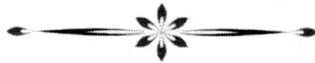

Calories per serving: 273
Yield: 1 Nutribullet cup - 24oz

Green Faith

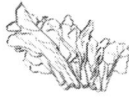

1 cup of Swiss chard, finely chopped
½ cup of watercress
1 cup of pineapple chunks
1 banana, sliced
1 cup of chilled green tea

Directions
Add the Swiss chard and watercress, followed by the pineapple and banana. Pour in the green tea and blend until smooth. Pour in some filtered water if more liquid is needed to reach the max line.

Health Benefits
Stimulates the release of digestive juices.
Regulates bowel movement.
Promotes healthy carbohydrate metabolism.
Reduces the risk of atherosclerosis, strokes, and heart disease.

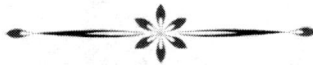

Calories per serving: 198
Yield: 1 Nutribullet cup - 24oz

Green Supreme

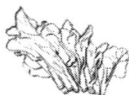

1 cup of romaine lettuce
1 cup of spinach
1 orange, peeled, pitted and cut into segments
1 red grapefruit, peeled, pitted and cut into segments
1 tablespoon of sesame seeds
1 cup of coconut water

Directions
Add the romaine lettuce and spinach, followed by the orange, grapefruit, and sesame seeds. Pour in the coconut water and blend until smooth. Add some filtered water if more liquid is needed to reach the max line.

Health Benefits
Helps to defend the body against bacterial and viral infections.
Improves sluggish blood circulation.
Helps to maintain healthy fluid balance in the body.
Lowers stress on the cardiovascular system.

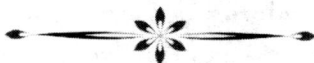

Calories per serving: 256
Yield: 1 Nutribullet cup - 24oz

Thriller Green

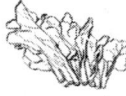

1 avocado
½ cup of parsley
1 cup of strawberries, finely chopped
1 teaspoon of bee pollen
1 teaspoon of manuka honey
Filtered water

Directions

Add the parsley, followed by the avocado, strawberries, bee pollen, and manuka honey. Pour in the filtered water to the max line and blend until smooth.

Health Benefits

Prevents the signs of premature aging.
Stimulates healthy digestion.
Increases healthy blood flow to organs and tissues of the body.
Helps to increase muscle tone.

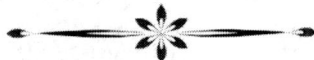

Calories per serving: 403
Yield: 1 Nutribullet cup - 24oz

Charming Green

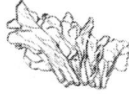

1 cup of dandelion greens, finely chopped
1 kiwi fruit, peeled
2 tangerines, peeled and pitted
½ cup of pitted cherries
Filtered water

Directions
Add the dandelion greens, followed by the kiwi fruit, tangerines, and cherries. Pour in the filtered water to the max line and blend until smooth.

Health Benefits
Helps to relieve congestion in the lungs and chest.
Reduces the risk of diarrhoea.
Reduces skin irritation.
Neutralises toxins in the body's cells.

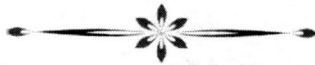

Calories per serving: 207.5
Yield: 1 Nutribullet cup - 24oz

West End Green

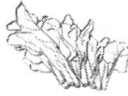

1 cup of collard greens
½ cucumber, sliced
1 celery stalk, sliced
1 mango, peeled and cored
Filtered water

Directions
Add the collard greens, followed by the cucumber, celery, and mango.
Pour in the filtered water to the max line and blend until smooth.

Health Benefits
Balances moods and helps to alleviate depression.
Maintains proper enzyme activity in the body.
Improves mental clarity and concentration.
Stimulates digestion.

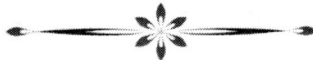

Calories per serving: 139.5
Yield: 1 Nutribullet cup - 24oz

A Green Lifetime

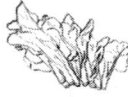

1 cup of arugula
1 cup of watercress
1 banana, sliced
2 peaches, pitted and chopped
½ teaspoon of cinnamon
Filtered water

Directions
Add the arugula and watercress, followed by the banana and peaches.
Sprinkle in the cinnamon and pour in the filtered water to the max
line. Blend until smooth.

Health Benefits
Protects against cardiovascular disease.
Provides relief from headaches and migraines.
Helps with healthy weight management.
Stimulates blood circulation.

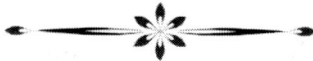

Calories per serving: 235
Yield: 1 Nutribullet cup - 24oz

Green Ghost

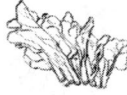

1 kiwi, peeled and chopped
1 apple, cored and chopped
1 pear, cored and chopped
1 lime, peeled and chopped
Filtered water

Directions
Add the kiwi fruit, apple, pear, and lime. Pour in the filtered water to the max line and blend until smooth.

Health Benefits
Promotes healthy bone mineral density.
Improves the transport of oxygen around the body.
Increases the strength of hair and nails.
Helps to regulate the production of hormones.

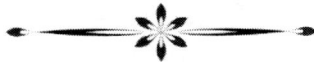

Calories per serving: 262
Yield: 1 Nutribullet cup - 24oz

Frenzy Green

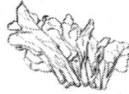

1 cup of collard greens, finely chopped
1 apple, cored and chopped
1 cup of strawberries, finely chopped
1 plum, pitted
1 tablespoon of ground flax seed
Filtered water

Directions
Add the collard greens, followed by the apple, strawberries, and plum. Sprinkle in the ground flax seed and pour in the filtered water to the max line. Blend until smooth.

Health Benefits
Improves bone and joint health.
Helps to prevent premature aging.
Stimulates healthy blood clotting.
Helps to reduce the growth of cancerous cells in the body.

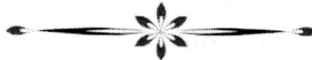

Calories per serving: 223
Yield: 1 Nutribullet cup - 24oz

Fade to Green

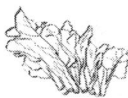

1 cup of dandelion greens, finely chopped
1 cup of pineapple chunks
1 passion fruit
1 banana, sliced
1 cup of chilled dandelion tea

Directions
Add the dandelion greens, followed by the pineapple, passion fruit, and banana. Pour in the dandelion tea, adding some filtered water if more liquid is needed to reach the max line. Blend until smooth.

Health Benefits
Helps to prevent the onset of type 2 diabetes.
Helps to lower high blood pressure.
Maintains healthy vision.
Helps to prevent constipation.

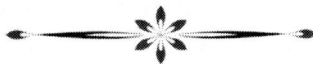

Calories per serving: 231
Yield: 1 Nutribullet cup - 24oz

The Green Whisperer

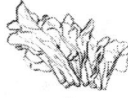

1 cup of arugula
1 red pepper, cored and sliced
1 green pepper, cored and sliced
½ cucumber, sliced
½ cup of crushed ice
Filtered water

Directions
Add the arugula, followed by the red and green peppers, the cucumber, and the ice. Pour in the filtered water to the max line and blend until smooth.

Health Benefits
Maintains healthy bone tissue.
Promotes the production of healthy enzymes.
Promotes healthy cell growth and development.
Stimulates collagen production.

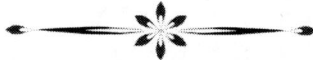

Calories per serving: 88.5
Yield: 1 Nutribullet cup - 24oz

Green Ga Ga

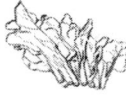

4 broccoli spears
1 cup of romaine lettuce
1 pear, cored and chopped
1 cup of raspberries
1 cup of chilled green tea

Directions
Add the romaine lettuce, followed by the broccoli, pear, and raspberries. Pour in the green tea, topping up with filtered water if more liquid is needed to reach the max line. Blend until smooth.

Health Benefits
Detoxifies the blood.
Helps to purify the kidneys and prevent kidney infections.
Increases metabolic activity in the body.
Boosts the immune system.

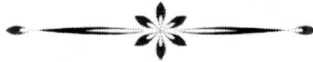

Calories per serving: 221
Yield: 1 Nutribullet cup - 24oz

Atomic Green

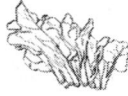

1 cup of kale leaves, finely chopped
2 carrots, peeled and sliced
2 kiwi fruit, peeled
Filtered water

Directions
Add the kale, followed by the carrots and kiwi fruit. Pour in the
filtered water to the max line and blend until smooth.

Health Benefits
Helps to lower high blood pressure.
Increases energy levels.
Increases nutrient uptake from food.
Helps to reduce bloating and fluid retention.

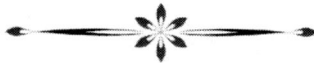

Calories per serving: 167
Yield: 1 Nutribullet cup - 24oz

Green Tropicana

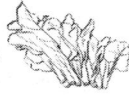

1 cup of Swiss chard, finely chopped
2 peaches, pitted
1 tangerine, peeled
½ grapefruit, cut into small segments
1 teaspoon of manuka honey
1 cup of coconut water

Direction
Add the Swiss chard, followed by the peaches, tangerine, grapefruit, and manuka honey. Pour in the coconut water, topping up with filtered water if more liquid is needed to reach the max line. Blend until smooth.

Health Benefits
Helps to balance cholesterol levels in the blood.
Increases bone health, helping to prevent osteoporosis.
Fights against inflammation in the body.
Stimulates the formation of new cells.

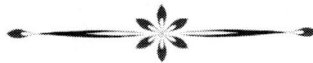

Calories per serving: 262
Yield: 1 Nutribullet cup - 24oz

The Green Countdown

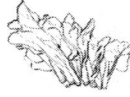

1 cup of spinach
1 cup of raspberries
1 cup of blueberries
1 cup of blackberries
1 tablespoon of goji berries
1 cup of coconut water

Directions
Add the spinach, followed by the raspberries, blueberries, blackberries, and goji berries. Pour in the coconut water, topping up with some filtered water if more liquid is needed to reach the max line.

Health Benefits
Boosts blood circulation.
Helps to prevent anaemia.
Stimulates moods and helps to alleviate depression.
Helps to prevent gastric ulcers.

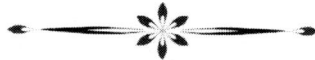

Calories per serving: 292
Yield: 1 Nutribullet cup - 24oz

Golden Green

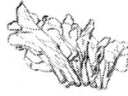

1 cup of collard greens
2 cups of watermelon chunks
½ cucumber, sliced
½ cup of crushed ice
Filtered water

Directions

Add the collard greens, followed by the watermelon, cucumber, and ice. Pour in the filtered water to the max line and blend until smooth.

Health Benefits

Helps to keep arterial walls strong and healthy.
Helps to eliminate blemishes from the skin.
Improves skin tone and elasticity.
Combats against colds and flu.

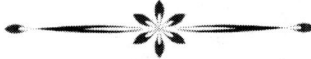

Calories per serving: 126.5
Yield: 1 Nutribullet cup - 24oz

Green Dove

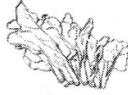

2 beets, peeled and chopped
1 orange, peeled and chopped
1 nectarine, pitted and chopped
1 teaspoon of spirulina
1 cup of chilled green tea

Directions
Add the beets, orange, and nectarine. Sprinkle in the spirulina and pour in the green tea, topping up with filtered water if more liquid is needed to reach the max line. Blend until smooth.

Health Benefits
Helps to reduce the build up of fat cells in the body.
Improves muscle strength.
Maintains the health of the nervous system.
Promotes the growth and development of tissue and cells.

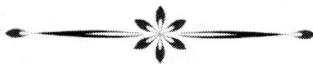

Calories per serving: 203
Yield: 1 Nutribullet cup - 24oz

The Green Star

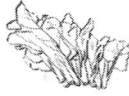

1 cup of collard greens, finely chopped
2 cups of strawberries
1 banana, sliced
1 tablespoon of cacao powder
1 cup of almond milk

Directions
Add the collard greens, strawberries, and banana. Sprinkle in the cacao powder and pour in the almond milk. Add some filtered water if more liquid is needed to reach the max line. Blend until smooth.

Health Benefits
Helps to maintain the cartilage in joints.
Supports hair growth.
Increases the transport of oxygen and nutrients around the body.
Accelerates the healing of wounds.

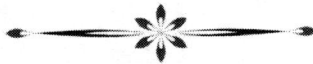

Calories per serving: 269
Yield: 1 Nutribullet cup - 24oz

Eternal Green

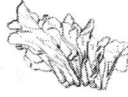

1 cup of watercress
1 cup of kale, finely chopped
1 cup of spinach
1 cup of romaine lettuce, finely chopped
2 apples, cored and chopped
Filtered water

Directions

Add the watercress, kale, spinach, and romaine lettuce, followed by the apples. Pour in the filtered water to the max line and blend until smooth.

Health Benefits

Stimulates collagen production in the body.
Helps to slow the aging process.
Helps to reduce the risk of cancer.
Maintains a healthy weight.

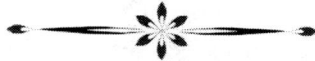

Calories per serving: 242
Yield: 1 Nutribullet cup - 24oz

The Green Reaction

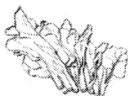

1 cup of dark green cabbage, finely chopped
1 cup of pitted cherries
1 orange, peeled, pitted and cut into segments
4 asparagus spears, sliced
Filtered water

Directions
Add the cabbage, followed by the cherries, orange, and asparagus.
Pour in the filtered water to the max line and blend until smooth.

Health Benefits
Reduces the risk for type 2 diabetes.
Helps to decrease bone loss.
Reduces the risk of coronary heart disease.
Aids in iron absorption.

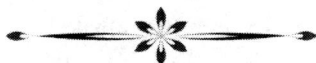

Calories per serving: 193
Yield: 1 Nutribullet cup - 24oz

Groovy Green

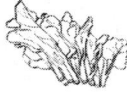

1 cup of spinach
1 cup of parsley, finely chopped
2 mint leaves
1 cup of green seedless grapes
1 kiwi fruit, peeled and chopped
1 tablespoon of ground almonds
Filtered water

Directions
Add the spinach, parsley, and mint leaves, followed by the grapes, kiwi fruit, and ground almonds. Pour in the filtered water to the max line and blend until smooth.

Health Benefits
Maintains a healthy blood pressure.
Regulates bowel movement.
Keeps the skin and eyes healthy.
Helps to reduce bad cholesterol levels.

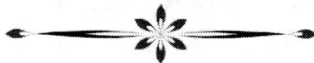

Calories per serving: 256
Yield: 1 Nutribullet cup - 24oz

The Green Gang

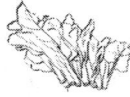

1 cup of romaine lettuce, finely chopped
1 cup of dandelion greens, finely chopped
1 cup of blackberries
1 cup of pineapple chunks
1 cup of chilled green tea

Directions
Add the romaine lettuce and dandelion greens, followed by the blackberries and pineapple chunks. Pour in the green tea, topping up with filtered water if more liquid is needed to reach the max line.

Health Benefits
Helps to form healthy blood cells.
Lowers the risk of heart disease.
Boosts the body's metabolic rate.
Increases energy levels.

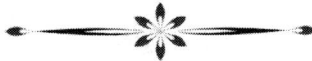

Calories per serving: 179
Yield: 1 Nutribullet cup - 24oz

References

Dr. Michael Murray & Dr. Joseph Pizzorno with Lara Pizzorno, MA, LMT, *The Encyclopaedia of Healing Foods.* Piatkus, 2006.

Nutribullet LLC, *Nutribullet User Guide & Recipe Book.*

Jonny Bowden, PhD., C.N.S., *The 150 Healthiest Foods on Earth.* Fair Winds Press, 2007.

Nutrient Data for ingredients listed was provided by USDA. *http://ndb.nal.usda.gov/ndb/foods*

CPSIA information can be obtained
at www.ICGtesting.com
Printed in the USA
FSOW02n2009281215
15061FS

9 781517 084523